THE LIFE AND TIMES
Of Papa Vark

THE MEMOIRS OF A CANCER SURVIVOR

WAYNE COOKE

ISBN: 1466327626

ISBN 13: 9781466327627

Dedication

This book is dedicated in memory of my parents, Gilbert and Lottie Cooke; to my devoted wife and caregiver, Patricia; in memory of my brother Dean; to my living siblings, Janet, Allen, Daniel and James; to my son Scott, his wife Cristina, and their three sons, Xavier, Rafael, and Felix; to my daughter Kelly, her husband Ante, and their son, Ante Wayne; to all of the family members, doctors and friends who have supported and strengthened me throughout my journey; and to cancer survivors everywhere.

Prologue

I am a cancer survivor. Stage IV colon cancer to be exact. The American Cancer Society publishes five year survival rates on many types of cancer and the cancer that I have has a five year survival rate of about 6-10%. So my odds are not too good, to say the least. On the other hand, in November of 2011 I will have survived for eight years, far beyond the expected survival rate.

After three major surgeries and over 130 sessions of infusion including five different chemo protocols, I am left with several pulmonary nodules in my lungs and a strange "something" on my liver. My oncologist, Dr. Peter Yi, tells me to treat my cancer as a chronic disease, to be treated and lived with but not cured. I will probably be on some sort of chemo for the rest of my life. But I seem to manage well.

Doctors are saying that I am unique, that I am one of a kind, that my case is remarkable and that I am a "Miracle Man." I don't have a good counter to those claims, other than to say that like the Mississippi, I just keep rolling along.

In 2007 and again in 2009, I worked on the story that became the book that was published in December 2009 entitled *On the Far Side Of the Curve: A Stage IV Colon Cancer Survivor's Journey.* In that book I described my then six-year journey in surviving colon cancer and included several anecdotes that I hoped would help explain why I had been successful up to then in my fight against the disease.

But as I thought about the stories to include in that book, I realized that there were many other interesting events in my life that might resonate with others and could be lost if I did not take the time to write them down. And it was actually in November 2009, on a New Jersey transit train home from an appointment at the Memorial Sloan-Kettering offices in NYC, that I started making a list of the possible chapters for this book. So I owe this book to my cancer. If I did not have cancer, I probably would not have been compelled to write this story and many of the events that you are going to read about in this book would have been lost.

My wife, Pat, then shared with me a book that she was reading that had many short chapters and I picked up on that approach as one that I could use effectively in this book. My objective was not to create a story that had a beginning and an end but to create a memoir of short vignettes that could each be read on their own merit.

I have also thought about the influence that my parents, particularly my father, have had on my life and have incorporated some of his guidance along the way. He was particularly forceful about using the skills that you have been given in life and not wasting them.

But why would anyone, other than my immediate family members, relatives and friends want to read this book? Well, for starters, many people just like to read biographies. And I submit that it is possible to gain insight from one person's life that may jog the memory of another- to give them some thoughts as to how they may have or may be able to lead their own lives. And there is value in doing that.

Then, in reference to the title, you might ask, "What is a Vark?" Regarding that question, I believe that it is significant enough to warrant a chapter of its own, and so that is where I will start.

CHAPTER 1
How I became Papa Vark!

I have had many nicknames over the years, but the most current one is Papa Vark.

It all started about 10 years ago. My daughter, Kelly, had graduated from Georgetown University with a degree in Languages and Linguistics, majoring in Mandarin. She was also interested in the evolving internet businesses and had moved into New York City to find her fame and fortune. Unfortunately, the company that she was working for around the Y2K timeframe went under, and she found herself living at home again, working on a local temp job until she could find something else in the city. It was about that time that the culture of the Varks was developed.

One day Kelly accused me of nosing around into her personal life, much in the style of an aardvark. Webster's New World dictionary defines an aardvark as "a nocturnal, ant-eating South African mammal" derived from the Dutch "earth pig."

I would have preferred to describe my activities more in the style of Sherlock Holmes' "a turn both for observation and for deduction" as described in Arthur Conan Doyle's *A Study in Scarlet*. But be that as it may, she chose to use the term aardvark which she shortened to just plain vark. In fact, over the years, I have received a number of variations of the name, including Lord Vark, King Vark, Chief Vark, Head Vark, but most often Papa Vark or simply PV.

She, in turn, named herself Baby Vark or BV, and when she moved to Hong Kong in 2007, she was "promoted" to Chief Asian Vark and her apartment there became "Vark Asian HQ."   Likewise, our home in Princeton, New Jersey became Vark International Headquarters, and in the summertime, Club Vark. You get the idea.

To round out the family organization, my wife, Pat, became Momma Vark or just MV, and our son was dubbed Frere Vark (Brother Vark in French), although the name did not really stick and he remained just plain Scott.

So the definitions PV, MV and BV have stuck over the years and you would frequently find them in use in family emails, on Christmas gift tags and on other types of correspondence. And in fact, I would submit that being defined as a vark implies that one is creative, intuitive, and, in most cases, intelligent, so it is a good thing to be recognized as a vark. It is a distinction to be treated with pride. And so Papa Vark just keeps on rolling.

CHAPTER 2
Two for the Price of One

I was born July 4, 1933 in Uniontown, Pennsylvania, where my father, Gilbert was a school teacher. A year later we moved to Madison, Wisconsin, where my father completed work on his Ph.D. in economics from the University of Wisconsin. I was told by my mother, Lottie, that one time during these early years, when I had gone out of the house to explore, she found me out by a fence talking to some cows. I trust that it was an intelligent conversation.

My earliest memories are from Grand Forks, North Dakota, where my father was teaching at a junior college. I can remember trying to avoid the tumbleweeds that used to blow through the streets. I was about three or four years old at the time and they were as big as I was.

In 1937 at the age of four, I remember being on the train as we went from Grand Forks to Bowling Green, Ohio where my father was going to be one of the first teachers at the business school that would later become Bowling Green State University. I was standing between two cars and almost fell off of the train until one of my parents grabbed me. If they had not been there at the right time, this could have been a very short book.

We first lived in a rental property at 508 South Main Street. I can remember sitting on the step as I waited for my older brother, Dean, to walk home from school, which was a couple of blocks up the street. He was two years older than I. I usually had my wagon with me so we could then go out and collect some of the buckeyes which were quite prevalent on the street where we lived. It is no wonder that Ohio is named "The Buckeye" State.

When I was about five years old my father, who was of the frugal type, had talked to a local doctor, Dr. Halleck, about doing a tonsillectomy on my brother, Dean. The interesting thing about it was that he was going to do it on our kitchen table with local lighting. As the time came for the procedure, someone, either my father or the doctor, suggested that since they were set up for the operation, they might as well do my tonsils at the same time. A "two-fer." So we got set up to do the operations in tandem, Dean first and then me. No problem, right?

Except that the electric power in our house went out. I don't know why or when it happened during the process. I do remember being told after the fact that they took my tonsils out by flashlight. So much for planning, and so much for hospital operations and problems with infections. But everything turned out ok. Dad got two tonsillectomies for the price of one. And Dean and I got a big dose of vanilla ice cream from Mom to help us recover. Homemade ice cream, of course.

CHAPTER 3
Fighting the "Japs"

December 7, 1941. It is Sunday afternoon, and Bill Urschel and I are lying on the living room floor of the home that my parents were renting at 318 North Summit Street in Bowling Green, Ohio listening to Bulldog Drummond on the radio. (We had moved to this house a couple of years earlier from the rental on South Main Street.) As was my normal function, I had my fingers wrapped around the antenna lead on the back of the radio to get better reception. The radio was a box type that you see in all of the '50s flashbacks. For whatever reason, my father had never attached an antenna cord to the radio, so I learned at an early age that to get decent reception I could put my thumb and forefinger on the antenna lead on the back of the radio and the reception improved.

Bill Urschel was a school chum who lived up the block on Summit Street and we became good friends over the years. Our family had grown to five children by now, four boys and a girl: Dean, Wayne, Janet, Allen and Dan, so we needed a larger house than the one on South Main Street. This house was conveniently located right across the street from the Ridge Street Elementary School, which I and my younger siblings all attended for six years.

Bill and I would listen to the radio a lot. There were a number of shows that would be on after school from 5 to 6 in the afternoon, including Jack Armstrong, Captain Midnight and The Lone Ranger, so it was a normal thing for us to be lying on the floor with the radio on.

This particular Sunday afternoon, Bill and I were listening to Bulldog Drummond when my older brother, Dean, burst into the room with some startling news. He had been spending the afternoon at the home of other friends, the Manharts. (Mr. Manhart was a business school professor who shared an office with my father at the University.) He had learned from them that the "Japs" had just bombed Pearl Harbor in Hawaii.

This was followed about an hour later by a paper boy in the street in front of our house shouting "Extra, Extra," with a special edition of the Toledo Blade announcing the attack. Bill went up the street to be with his family, and Dean and I discussed what we were going to do next.

———————

Over the next few years, we got involved in a lot of war-related activities, including working with "Spot a Plane" cards (to identify any Japanese Zero fighters or Mitsubishi Bombers that flew our way), making model airplanes, and converting the vacant lot next to the Manharts house into a series of trenches. There we practiced our war games so we could be ready for any attack.

We were more worried about the Japanese coming from the Pacific than the Germans coming from Europe, since we expected the British to help hold the Nazis at bay in the Atlantic. And we were well equipped. Besides our Spot-a-Plane cards, we had battle maps and kept track of all of the activities of the war. A group of us got together at Steve McEwen's house across town and made models of airplanes of all types. One that I made was a B29 Bomber with camouflage paint. I thought that it was really neat and I had it for years.

And what we did obviously worked, since the "Japs" never did get as far as Bowling Green, Ohio.

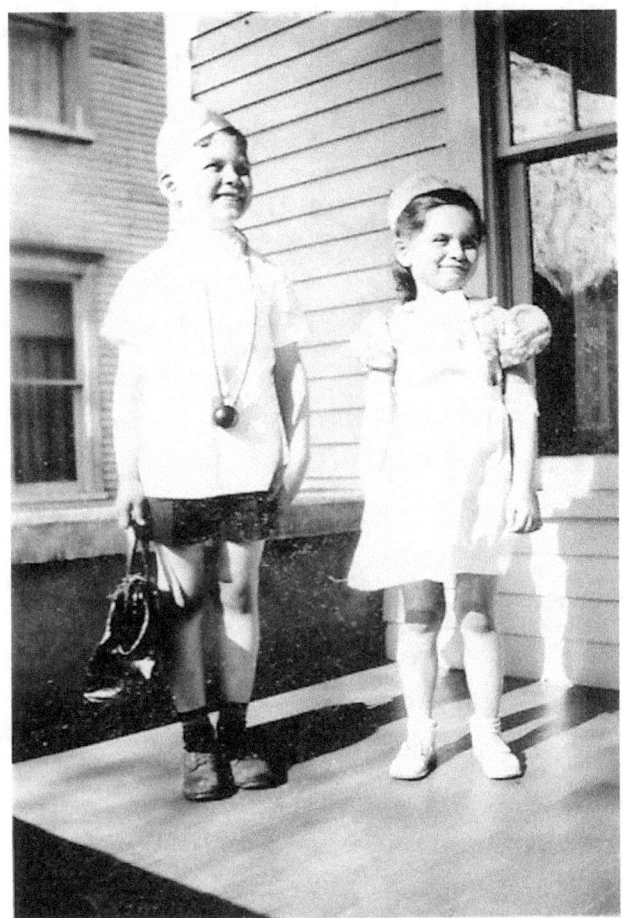

With Janet at 318 North Summit St

CHAPTER 4
Football on the School Yard/School Patrol

Bill Urschel had an older brother, Hal, who we held in high regard. He was a year older than Dean and was good at just about everything. When Bill and I were in elementary school and Dean and Hal were in Junior High, we used to play a lot of touch football on the front lawn of the Ridge Street School. Bill and I were on one team and Hal and Dean on the other. We would touch them and they would tackle us.

We had a lot of good games there and used the flag pole and the trees on the lawn strategically. One of our key plays was "straight down the sideline, and then cut past the big tree and go down around the flagpole." Later on, the school made us stop using the front lawn and instead use the playground in the back of the school. It was ok, but not as much fun as the front lawn: no trees and no flagpole.

―――――――――

We had a student-run school patrol at the Ridge Street School that operated before and after school to help the younger students make the crossings at four streets. Normally the school patrol was comprised of sixth-grade students. For some reason, when I was in the fifth grade, they needed more students for the patrol. I was chosen and spent two years as captain of the school patrol. I soon became expert on going into the street to stop the cars to let the students cross. Probably today, they would do it differently.

––––––––––––––––––

My first exposure to Princeton, New Jersey, was through Hal Urschel. He had a scholarship to Princeton University and played football there, and he was pretty good at it. At that time, Princeton seemed like the end of the world for someone like me who had not been east of Northwestern Ohio since the age of one. But Hal played first-string guard on the Princeton National Championship team of 1950 and at his home up the street, I met a number of the Princeton players including Dick Kazmaier, who lived in nearby Maumee, Ohio, and won the Heisman Trophy in 1951. I was in awe. Little did I know at that time that 24 years later I would be moving to Princeton with IBM.

CHAPTER 5
Sharing a Paper Route with Dean

My older brother Dean was two years older than I was, but he had skipped a grade along the way so he was three years ahead of me in school. Therefore, when I was in the fourth grade, he was in the seventh. About that time he decided to get a paper route delivering the Toledo Blade to a route that was adjacent to and included Bowling Green State University.

Delivery was six days a week, including weekdays and Saturdays. Saturday morning you made the rounds to collect. As I remember, the cost of delivery was $.27 a week per paper, and the delivery boy got $.03 of the cost. So with a route of 50 customers, you would make $1.50 per week. To put that in context, the cost of the Saturday afternoon matinee at the Lyric Theater was about $.14. An ice cream cone or a bottle of coke was about a nickel.

After a while, Dean got so busy with school activities, such as football practice, that in order to make sure that deliveries would be on time each day, he enlisted me to help him out. Dean decided that it would be fair to divide the proceeds 60/40, so his share of our weekly paper route income was $.90 per week and my share was $.60. This was an early real world experience for me in dealing with fractions.

I don't remember how we divided up the delivery, but I do remember loading up my paper bag, lugging the bag over my shoulder, getting on my bicycle and cycling out to the University to deliver the papers. As Dean got more involved with activities at school, he got less interested in the paper route, and when he turned sixteen he started working at the local Kroger Store. At some point in time, I took over the whole responsibility and got the whole proceeds, not just forty percent.

A store in downtown Bowling Green called Rappaports sold all sorts of stuff that kids would like. One thing that I liked was a cardboard cutout of a train engine. You punched out the pieces and then put the engine together. It would have been about the size of a shoe box when put together and it sold for twenty five cents. I did not get an allowance at that time, but I can remember badgering my mother for the money to buy that engine. She never relented and somehow I had managed to do without it. A lesson in frugality. But now that I had the paper route, I could make my own decisions on how I spent my own money.

One time I threw a paper through a customer's front window. I confessed to the homeowner and told him that I would pay him back for getting the window fixed. As I remember, it took almost forever to save up the money to pay him.

At about the same time, my friend Bill Urschel got an ice-cream cart route that included the University. We would meet up in the afternoon at the football practice field where the Cleveland Browns with coach Paul Brown, Otto Graham, Lou Groza, Marion Motley, et al were having their pre-season football camp. We would watch the practice for a while, and when the team took a break, Bill would ring the bell on his cart and sell ice-cream to the onlookers. Then I would continue on to deliver the papers. It was fun to get together with Bill in the middle of a hot summer's afternoon.

One of my customer's homes was located behind the University, down past the cemetery and I had to bike quite a ways to get to that house. I was always nervous going past the cemetery and would peddle as fast as I could to get down and back without seeing any ghosts or vampires. Today the university has totally built up the land around the cemetery so it doesn't seem nearly so threatening as it once did.

I used my paper route earnings to support my hobbies of collecting stamps and comic books. I would get stamps on approval from companies like H.E. Harris and the Mystic Stamp Company and started on a worldwide collection. My son, Scott, and I picked up collecting again when we lived in Paris with visits to the Marche Au Timbre (Stamp Market). We set up the Dad & Lad Stamp Collection (D & L) that concentrated on early United States stamps from 1847 on. But over time, Scott started focusing more on his collection of baseball cards. So I now have all of the stamp albums and the memories as well.

I also had some early Superman comic books but, for some reason, I sold off my collection before the Superman comics became so valuable. Little did I know.

CHAPTER 6
Christmas Shopping in Toledo

My dad owned a 1937 Chevrolet that you needed to crank to start. Sometimes it took several tries to get it going. In 1944 my youngest brother, Jim, was born and the Cookes became a family of eight with six kids, Dean, Janet, me, Al, Dan, and Jim. We had to get well organized to get all of us in the car. Wartime rationing was in force, so we needed coupons to buy gasoline and tires. We did not use the car that often. But our parents often decided that we needed a break from the limitations of shopping in Bowling Green, so at Christmas time we started going to Toledo, located 24 miles to the north, on an annual trek around Thanksgiving to have a day of shopping in the larger stores located there.

But the first question was how to get eight people in the car? Well my Dad, Gilbert, drove, of course. For some reason my Mom, Lottie, had learned to drive but never did. Mom sat in the front passenger seat holding Jim. One of the little guys, Al or Dan, would sit in the middle of the front and Dean, Janet and I would bring up the back seat with the other little brother on Dean's lap. No seatbelts in those days. We would drive up to Toledo at the 35 mph speed limit.

Then we would divide up into two groups, one with Mom and one with Dad, so no one would get lost and also so the one group would not know what the family members of the other group had purchased. We were assigned a modest allowance toward the cost of our purchases.

Mom always liked to start at a store called Lasalles. She was the most fun to go with, so I always tried to start with her. Off we would go with a time set for us to re-convene again at the car for the trip back. It all worked out pretty well and was a good lesson in family sharing. And it was also fun opening the presents on Christmas Day.

CHAPTER 7
"Doc" Cooke

My father, Gilbert, was a professor in the college of Business Administration at Bowling Green State University, one of the first two business school professors to be hired. Mr. Lewis Manhart was the other. Dad was very well respected and liked by his students and probably one of the most intelligent individuals that I have ever known.

In the mid 1940s, after Jim was born, Dad bought his first house at 445 North Prospect Street about two blocks from our rental house on North Summit, and also across the street from the Ridge Street School. This house was not far from the large playground behind the school building where we played touch football.

It was still a reasonable walk to the University campus, and most mornings he would leave the house early if he had an 8AM class. So even in the winter, which could get rather cold and snowy in Northwestern Ohio, he would pull on his Daniel Boone type cap and make that walk, whistling as he went. Gas and tires were rationed, so he used the car as little as possible and normally kept it in the detached garage next to the house.

He was a man of small stature, about 5' 6," but he had large brainpower. To put it bluntly, he was smart. He did not flaunt that skill, but after talking to him for a while, you knew that he had it and you did not want to take him on in that department.

He also worked his tail off for his family. When he was not teaching at the University, he was working as a sales clerk in the hardware department at the local Montgomery Wards store, keeping books for various businesses in town, working at the local Heinz plant, or doing whatever else he could to use his skills to make money to support his family. After he passed away, we found one of his budget books in the papers in his desk, and he had kept track of almost every nickel that he had earned and spent in supporting the eight Cookes. I guess I know where I learned that trick from.

When he worked at Montgomery Wards, he would often bring home one of their catalogs which my siblings and I would peruse just in case Santa might need some suggestions. Catalogs in those days were used almost as much as a dictionary. Today they have been generally replaced by the internet.

During my senior year in high school, he hired Bill Urschel and me to help dig out the unfinished part of our basement at the house at 445 N. Prospect. My parents turned part of the new basement into a bedroom and bathroom for college student renters and part into a playroom and a place for Dad to work on his various projects. After dinner, he would often go to the basement to work on one of the various school text books that he wrote, typing away on the Remington upright typewriter well into the night.

If he was not doing that, he was probably out at a meeting of the various committees he served on: PTA, School Board, Town Planning Commission, Sigma Alpha Epsilon fraternity advisors, Boy Scouts, Cub Scouts, etcetera. You name it, and he was probably on it. He never ran for a town office, unless you call being president of the PTA an elected official, but if he had, he probably could have won since most people in town knew who he was and thought highly of him. He did not have a political affiliation, but called himself an independent. He said that he voted for whom he thought was the best candidate, not based on party affiliation. He was raised an Episcopalian but since there was no Episcopal church in town, he joined Mom in going to the Methodist church.

Dad helped out many organizations in town over the years but the last thing that he would do is "blow his own horn." His rationale, I am sure, was that if you had the talent to do something, you had an obligation to others to use it where needed. Don't waste it. Kind of like the plaque that one of my IBM managers had on his wall that said "There is no limit to what can be accomplished if it does not matter who gets the credit." Gilbert personified that statement.

But there was one person in town that he could not stand-a certain lawyer. Dad said he was only out to build his own image and took any credit that he could, whether deserved or not. Any time this lawyer got any publicity or advertised or was written up for anything in the papers, Dad would stomp around and criticize him. While Dad almost refused to take any credit on his own, he was equally against any others who did, particularly if he did not think it was deserved.

I am not sure if it happened when Dad was alive or not, but sometime after I left town, a new brick and stone building was built on Main Street. It was a law office with this lawyer's name etched in stone across the front. I don't know if Dad ever knew about it, but if he did he would have turned over in his grave.

Shortly before he retired from the Bowling Green State University Business School, the school did a survey of the students to find out who they considered to be the five most respected teachers of all time. Gilbert Cooke was on the list. Most of the students who attended the school from 1937 to 1969 probably had fond memories of "Doc" Cooke.

One interesting fact about Dad was that during the summers, he often worked at the Heinz tomato ketchup plant that was located about four blocks from our house. One summer in the '40s, there were a number of German prisoners of war assigned there. (Yes, the war had found its way to Bowling Green.) Dad was working at the plant that summer, and when we asked him what he was doing there. he casually mentioned that he was translating for the prisoners.

What we kids hadn't ever focused on (or at least I had not) was that he was raised in Rochester, Minnesota, in the middle of a German community and his mother was of German descent (as were both of Mom's parents). They had spoken German in the home before the First World War, so he knew German. During the First World War, most of those families refrained from speaking German so people would not get suspicious of their intentions. In any case when called upon, Dad brought back his German and put it to use talking to the prisoners. It was a talent he had that we never would have thought about.

He also liked the Detroit Tigers. In his later years, you could frequently find him sitting in his favorite chair with a radio plugged into his ear, listening to Ernie Harwell and the ball game on WJR Radio.

Thinking back on it, he was an amazing person and used his talents to the fullest. I appreciate him a lot more now than I did then.

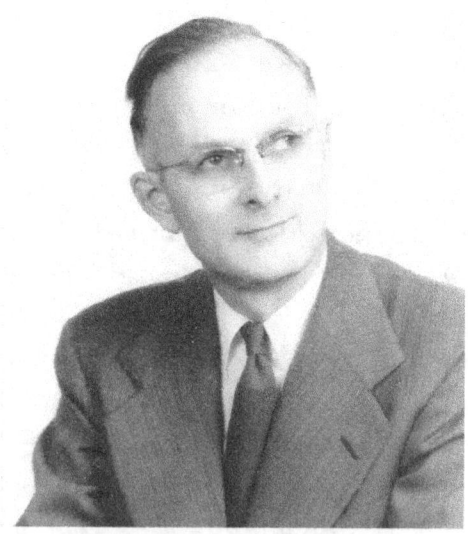

Gilbert "Doc" Cooke

CHAPTER 8
Life in Bowling Green

There were a number of kids in our neighborhood in Bowling Green, Ohio of about the same ages. What we learned early on was that with a bicycle you could get to any place in town. We could walk to the Lyric Theater on West Wooster Street, so you didn't need a bicycle for that. pay your $.14 and watch the news, the cartoon, the serial and the western. But if Dad wanted me to go to our "Victory Garden" which was located near the University past Manhart's house on Crim Street to hoe the carrots, beans, potatoes, etcetera, well, I needed a bicycle. And it helped to bicycle to the junior high or the high school, although I could walk it if I needed to. So the bicycle was my preferred method of transportation all through the school years.

One of our preferred games was rubber guns. We would make the gun from a couple of pieces of wood, and add a separate piece of wood, preferably a clothes pin, as the lever on the back. You would make your rubber "bullet" from a thin strip of inner-tubing that you would make a knot in and you were good to go. Insert the loose ends of the rubber "bullet" into the lever and pull the closed end over the end of the gun. It was preferable to use red pre-war inner-tubes whenever possible. The black synthetic rubber inner-tubes made during the war did not stretch as well and were to be avoided.

By putting lower pressure on the lever, the rubber bullet was released and fired to its target, probably one of the kids on the other side of whatever the teams were. It was only after a couple of kids suffered some nasty welts from the "bullets" that some of the moms called a moratorium on the rubber guns.

We also had a couple of nasty spells of polio in town. The community pool would be closed, and at least once the town was quarantined. We would be limited to playing on our city block- could not cross any street. Fortunately, I had friends living on the block, including one of my school classmates, Chuck Young, who lived a few houses down the street, so the quarantine was not as damaging to our fun as it could have been.

But in the fall of my senior year in high school, one of my good friends, Jim Kreischer, whom I had gone to Buckeye Boys State with the previous year, developed polio and became paralyzed from the neck down. He was on a rocking-cradle type breathing machine 24/7. They would set up a book on a stand in front of him and he developed a technique where he could turn the pages by putting pressure on his chin. One time, a year out of high school, a small group of friends and I went to see him and sang a modified version of "Carol of the Bells" to lift his spirits. But the disease got the better of him and he died two years later.

It was some time after our high school days that polio vaccines were developed and the disease was conquered. Several others of my high school classmates, including Jim Sherer and Jack Clark also suffered from polio. During our school days, it was a continual source of concern.

Few kids had cars at that time. One of my friends, Ollie Kaetzel, who lived a block or so up the street, got a car in his senior year, and on cold winter days would often stop to pick me up.

So life in Bowling Green was pretty normal for small-town Ohio, and we did have the University that added a number of activities, including sports events. As kids we made up a lot of our own games and also made do when we had to deal with the problems of the day, like polio.

CHAPTER 9
445 North Prospect

445 North Prospect was the family home from 1944 to 1967, when our parents moved to a one floor ranch house on Ranch Court over near the community park. By that time, Gilbert had suffered a heart attack and a couple of small strokes so they wanted a smaller house with a first floor master bedroom. But 445 was the house that we all lived in through junior high and high school.

It had two porches in the front of the house, one upstairs and one downstairs. Great for sitting in the swing or the rocking chairs on a humid summer's night. On the first floor there was a large entry hall, a front parlor room, where we had the piano for Janet to play, a living room, dining room, kitchen (with ice-box) and back hall with a powder room.

On the second floor, it originally had four bedrooms. Dean and I shared the front bedroom that faced Prospect Street. Mom and Dad had the middle bedroom, facing Crim Street. Dan and Al had the third bedroom, behind Mom and Dad's, and Janet had a small bedroom across the hall that included a stairway to the attic. There was one full bathroom with a tub and no shower at the end of the hall. Jim was in a crib when we moved into the house, and later Dad worked with a neighbor to convert a small loft space on the second floor for a bedroom for Jim. It all worked out ok.

The basement had a large coal furnace that Dad had to stoke up every night during the winter. After Bill Urschel and I helped Dad in digging out the basement, he converted the coal furnace to a gas one, and Jim took over the coal bin for a chemistry lab which he furnished with used equipment Dean acquired from The Ohio State University, where he was majoring in chemistry at the time..

There are many stories to be told about the house on North Prospect. It was really special at holidays such as Christmas when Mom would make sure that the place was well decorated and enjoyable.

In the back yard we had a large cherry tree with some low hanging limbs that for many years was used for climbing. It was a part of all of our childhoods. We had a large side yard, big enough for a touch football game for four, two on a side. However, the house had curved windows in the living room and some 220 volt wires along that side of the house. Dad was always concerned that someone would break one of the windows or hit the 220s, although no one ever did.

I believe that all of us had fond memories of 445 North Prospect.

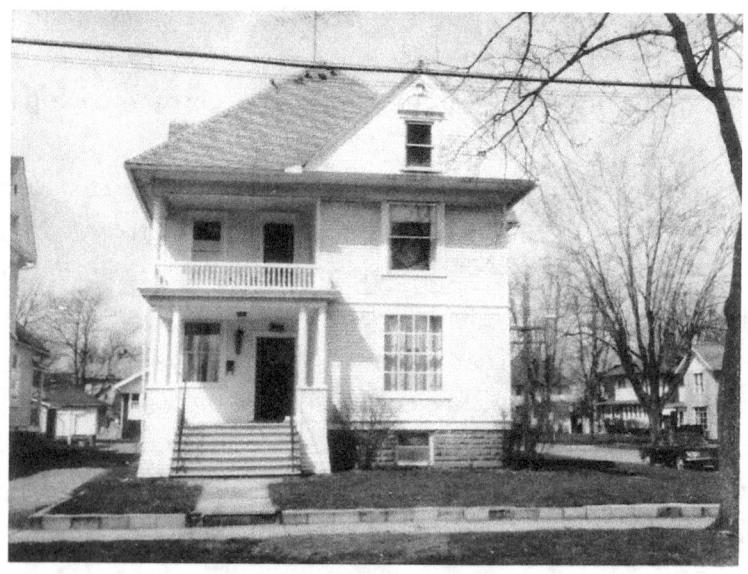

445 North Prospect Street

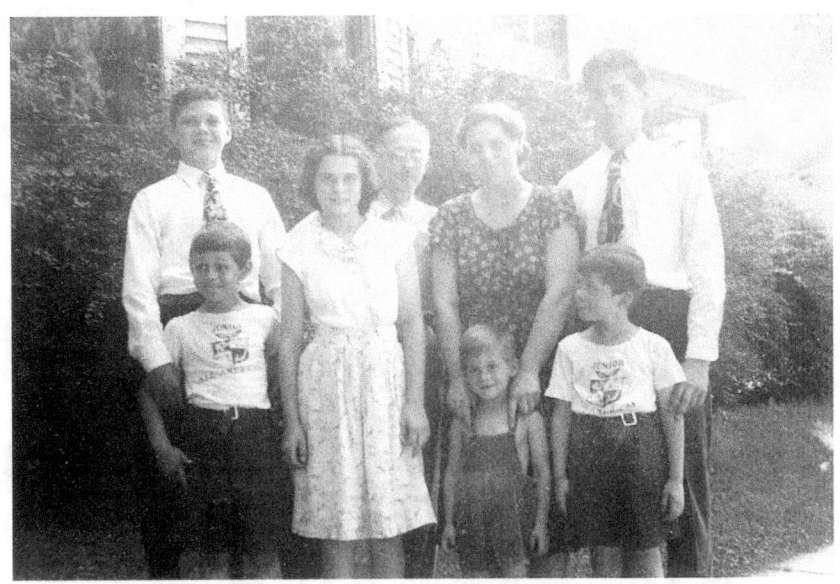

Cooke Family at 445 N. Prospect Street, Circa 1948

CHAPTER 10
Technology

Some of the biggest changes in our lives over the past fifty years have been the increase and diversity in the use of technology, and I have been eyeball to eyeball with a number of the changes. Five technologies that are of particular interest are the telephone, the television, the stereo, the typewriter and the computer.

When I was growing up in Ohio, we had one phone in the house -in the kitchen, of course- and it was on a party line. What that meant was that there were two houses, ours and the one next door, which had the same phone number. If we wanted to make a call, we had to ring up the operator, give her the number to be called and have her place the call. If we were to receive a call, the operator would give one ring on the phone for our house and two rings on the phone if it was for the house next door. If we got one ring, we would know to pick up the phone since the call was for us. Mom taught all of us phone etiquette. If I picked up the phone I was to say, "Cooke's residence, Wayne speaking." And so on, for the rest of the family.

My dad never did trust our next door neighbor and frequently made the accusation to the family that he was listening in on our conversations, which one could do with the party line if one were so inclined. Dad said that he could hear him breathing on the phone. I am not sure of what value listening in on our conversations would be, but it was possible although we never proved it. As you might imagine, any long distance calls were very exceptional and only done in limited number. And cell phones and smart phones were way off in the distance.

We were probably one of the last homes in Bowling Green to get a television- at least the last among my friends. Dad thought that we could make better use of our time than by watching stuff on the "tube." Television started to get more popular when I was in high school, so if I wanted to watch anything, like Milton Berle, I had to go over to one of my friend's houses.

I had two friends within walking distance with TVs: Bill Urschel, who lived a block up Summit Street, and Bennett Litherland, who lived a couple of blocks away across Main Street. So If I wanted to watch a particular show, I would normally see one of them at school and schedule a visit.

Watching TV during the '50s reminds me of the opening of the Simpsons: everyone crowding around the TV set in the living room. When I visited one of them, particularly Bennett, his parents would be there and we would all gather in the living room for the "main event." There was usually no more than one TV per household in those days and it was in black and white with a rabbit-ear antenna. It was a while before color television made its appearance.

We didn't have a record player in our house until I was a junior in high school. I know because I bought a table-top player that year with money from my job at the local Kroger store. I had started working in the Kroger store bagging groceries at $.65 per hour when I turned sixteen, following in the footsteps of my older brother, Dean. I later advanced to working with produce and at the check-out and even had a short stint in the meat department. The money was good for a high school kid, although the hours conflicted with a number of school activities.

I particularly did not like working on Friday night, which during the school year was often a basketball game followed by a school dance. But Friday night was also a busy time at the Kroger store. The store closed at 9PM and I often worked until 10 and then went to the high school dance after the game in my white work shirt. It was probably a little sweaty, but that was the way it was. I did take the bow tie off.

In any case, I had my own money which I was saving primarily for college, but I did go after the record player. It was a table-top device with no changer, but boasted three speeds; 78 rpm, 33 1/3 rpm, and when you added the disk adapter, 45 rpm. I liked music and started buying records of all types, both pop and classical. One particularly interesting purchase I made was a grab bag of classical music from the Wards catalog. It was a potpourri of RCA red seal 12" records: the gold standard of the day. You had no choice in the pieces but it was a very interesting collection and sparked my interest in classical music. I believe that I kept the record player and my collection downstairs so the family could enjoy it as well.

My father used an old Remington upright typewriter to write his text books for the University. As I remember, one of the most difficult tasks was making corrections. There were no copiers in those days so if you wanted to create a typed page with copies, you would have to back the original sheet with carbon paper between each of the other sheets of paper. If you wanted to make a correction, you had to take the whole stack of papers out and then erase the mistake page by page. Insert the pages again, line them up and hope that when you typed the corrections they ended up in the right spot. It was a very tedious process, very prone to error, and one that I became very familiar with when I was typing college papers on my Underwood portable.

And as for computers, the primary method of processing data in the '50s was the punched card. The personal computer was three decades away, and the electronic computer had not yet reached any type of expanded use but was for business use only at the time. I will get more into computers when we talk a bit about my days at IBM.

––––––––––––––––––

The changes in technology are some of the most dramatic changes that we have experienced in life over the past fifty years. As I sit here at my wireless laptop and then read in the newspapers about all of the new media and personal devices, I realize that the last fifty years were just the introduction to many more technology changes to come. I hope that my inquisitive nature is up to the task.

Of course Mother Nature can interrupt all of this with a storm like the one we had on the East Coast in August 2011 that takes all of the power and the phone lines out and makes us revert to candles (and flashlights) for several days. We can then better appreciate how Washington and Jefferson must have lived.

CHAPTER 11
Boy Scouts/Camp Miakonda

Dad was the scoutmaster of Boy Scout troop 338. It was sponsored by the First Methodist Church but had members from all over town. I was an active member, and had also been active in Cub Scout Pack 338 that was the "minor league" feeder for the troop with boys from 8-11 years old. By now the rules have changed a bit, but in those days the Boy Scouts were primarily 12-15 years old and were generally in the seventh to ninth grades.

One of the requirements for advancement was the fourteen-mile hike. Normally you would take the hike in the summer time, probably with the other members of your patrol of about five to seven other scouts. You would hike to a location about seven miles away that had facilities for cooking, and nature hikes. There you would spend some leisure time and eventually make your trip back and qualify for the event.

I did not do it in the normal way. For some reason, I decided to do the hike on a bitter cold day in winter. I probably had to get it done to qualify for some achievement level. But I do not remember why and I did not plan do it with my patrol but by myself. I was going to walk to a town about seven miles north of Bowling Green and then turn around and walk back. So I bundled myself up and, against the arguments of my mother, started out.

I was a few miles into the walk when I noticed someone coming up on the road behind me. It was my brother, Dean. He caught up with me and said that Mom had asked him to do the walk with me to make sure that I did ok. So we walked together up to the neighboring town and then made our turn to walk back. It was really cold. Several cars stopped to find out if we needed any help or a ride back to town, which we declined.

After we had walked about halfway back, Dean said that he was sure that I could handle the rest of the hike by myself and, since he was getting cold, started on ahead. I was walking as fast as I could, given the cold conditions, but he wanted to walk even faster, and I let him go.

I eventually made it home and completed the requirement for the fourteen mile hike. I am not sure if it was a testament to my determination or my stupidity, but as far as the fourteen mile hike went, I had checked it off of my list.

One of the fun things about becoming a Boy Scout was that you were eligible to go the Boy Scout camp in nearby Sylvania, Ohio, called Camp Miakonda. I started going to the camp when I was 12 years old. They had lots of fun stuff- a lake for boating and canoeing, a large swimming pool, trails for bird watching. Camp crafts, a trading post where you could buy craft supplies and things, a big dining hall for mess call and a large outdoor Indian style arena for a pow-wow gathering of all of the scouts attending camp that week.

There were also various types of camp sites- an Indian village with teepees, tent camps, tree houses, and, where we most often stayed, Adirondack style structures with roofs and floors and tent-type walls sleeping about 8 scouts each. Each troop was assigned a village location, which had enough space for 20-30 scouts and a common area in the middle.

During the week you could work on a variety of merit badges and skills, as well as participate in recreational activities. When we were at camp, Dad was the leader of our troop and looked very Boy Scoutish dressed up in his camp garb. A number of my friends from school, including Bill Urschel and Carl Helms, were members of the troop. My older brother, Dean, had been a member of the troop, but because he was three years ahead of me in school, he was rarely at the camp at the same time. I worked hard at getting through the various merit badges and was pretty good in the aquatic skills. By the time I was 15 I had qualified for the swimming, lifesaving, rowing and canoeing merit badges and had achieved the rank of Eagle Scout.

Between the ninth and tenth grade, I worked at the Trading Post in the camp selling craft supplies, candy and other essentials. I also worked as a lifeguard. Three of us including my school classmate, Carl Helms, who was the senior member of the trading post staff, and Jerry Hawley, the camp bugler, shared a cabin for the summer. I had a budget book and kept track of all of the money that I spent throughout the summer- every nickel.

I remember that over the summer my bathing suit got a little worn and I wanted to get a new one. But I could not afford it so I found a bathing suit in the camp Lost and Found, washed it up and used it for the rest of the summer. I did not tell my mom about it because I knew that she would not approve.

Carl and I also continued our quest to learn to play bridge. At the scout camp, Carl, Jerry and I would find a fourth and set up at a table in our cabin when we weren't working at the Trading Post. It was a fun experience.

In my first book *On the Far Side of the Curve,* I tell the story of making a stab at being one of the two camp buglers that summer. That did not work out so well for me. I made a better effort at working at the Trading Post, lifeguarding and learning to play bridge.

Carl's parents liked to play bridge and on a Sunday afternoon, I would frequently walk the four blocks to their house on Crim Street in Bowling Green, where we would listen to classical music, and Carl and I would take on his parents in a few hands. I was then able to work on love of music and bridge playing at the same time.

CHAPTER 12
Roy V. Hilty, Chorale Director

Roy Hilty was the director of our junior high and senior high school choruses, and I sang under his direction for six years. You had to audition to get into the choruses, and he would hold small group sessions where you learned to read music and to work on tonality, pitch and other musical skills. So the choruses were pretty good. I sang tenor all through junior high and into my sophomore year of high school. At the time they were short on tenors in the Methodist Church choir, so I was drafted to sing tenor there as well. My voice changed by the end of my sophomore year, however, and for the rest of high school I was singing bass.

Both the junior and the senior high choruses would do a Christmas concert and other performances throughout the school year. Perhaps the most fun was when we would get on the school busses and go to another school for a joint concert or go to Toledo or somewhere else for a larger gathering of choruses. Our high school could not always compete with the neighboring schools on the athletic field, but we could compete in singing. We looked forward to the competitions because we knew that we were good.

It was under Mr. Hilty's direction that I first worked seriously on my musical skills. I learned to read music, sing better and learn some of the choral repertoire.

In both junior and senior high, I was quite busy in school activities outside of sports. In addition to singing, I was in dramatic groups, student council, honor society, announcement team, etcetera-just about anything that did not require athletic ability. And I loved reading. In Junior High it was fictional books like the Hardy Boys (which I still have, by the way, in my basement.) But in Senior High I shifted to non-fiction, particularly biographies, ancient history and American revolutionary war stuff. I still enjoy reading today.

It was at the commencement exercise to graduate from ninth grade that I received the American Legion award to honor the outstanding male graduating student. The girl who also won the award was Virginia Anderson, who had been my first date for a movie at the Cla-zel Theater a few years previously. She was now dating a three-sport athlete.

I am sure that Gilbert was quietly very proud of his #2 son. And I felt pretty good about using my skills.

CHAPTER 13
The River Horse

After I purchased my first record player, one of the albums that I bought was "Bozo at the Circus." I thought my younger brothers would enjoy it. They were ages 10, 9 and 6 at the time. One of my several nicknames would evolve from that album. The album tells the story of Bozo the Clown going to visit a number of animals at the circus; the Chimpanzee, the Elephant, etcetera and the animals describe the various aspects of their lives. One animal he visited was the hippopotamus or "River Horse." The hippo would describe his life very slowly in a very low voice.

Over time I was able to quote the hippo almost verbatim, and so to my younger brothers I became the "River Horse." To this day I am frequently asked to re-live the River Horse dialogue to nieces, nephews, and now grandchildren. Would you believe, a River Horse Brewery has opened up on the Delaware River about 15 miles from our family home, and River Horse Ale is now available at local liquor stores. Tastes pretty good.

I am actually pretty proud to be called "The River Horse."

The River Horse (hippopotamus) dialogue goes like this: (Slowly in a low voice).

"I'm always tired, it seems.
If you had my weight to carry around, you'd be tired too.(pause)

In Africa, I'm called the River Horse.
I like to stand in the mud of the rivers.(pause)
I'm about the biggest thing around here!
Gosh, I'm sleepy."

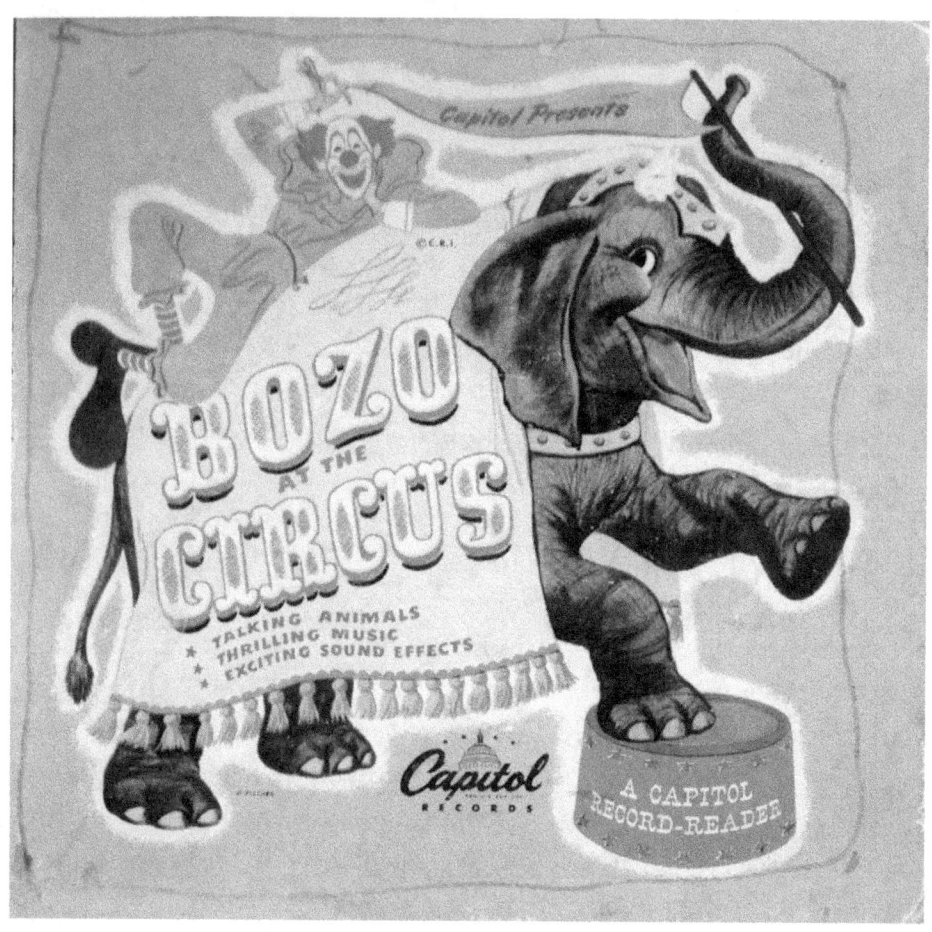

"Bozo at the Circus"

CHAPTER 14
Lottie

While my father, Gilbert, was the quiet motivator of the Cooke family, my mother, Lottie, was the glue that held everything together. Gilbert left the raising of the family to her. She cooked, she baked, she cleaned, and she washed the clothes and the dishes-everything that was needed to keep the family of eight going. We always had clean clothes, even if they might have been hand-me-downs. And as one of eight children in a Zumbro Falls, Minnesota German farm family, she had a good background for the job.

Traditions that she probably developed during her childhood, she passed down to her children. First, Sunday was the day to go to church. On Sunday she would make sure that each of her six children were well dressed, and then we would walk the four blocks to the Methodist Church where the eight of us filled up one of the pews.

After church we would have a family dinner, typically roast beef, mashed potatoes with gravy, vegetables and dessert. We would often have a student or visitor at the table to share the meal. After the meal, the kids would be divided up to clear, wash and wipe the dishes. We did not have an electric dishwasher and did it all by hand. We also did not have a refrigerator but for many years relied on an ice box with periodic visits from the ice man, who would deliver a block of ice for the upper box.

Lottie also made sure that we properly celebrated the holidays and birthdays, many times at picnics with the Manharts or the Helms. We would often spend the Fourth of July at Helms' house where we would party in their back yard and then sit on top of their garage to watch the fireworks at the local park. It was also my birthday so it was a special occasion.

Lottie had good genes and hopefully passed them on to her children. While Gilbert had more of a frail build and passed away just past their 50th wedding anniversary in 1976 when he was just 76, Lottie lived to be 94. Well into her '80s she was teaching crafts to the women in the "old-folks home." She had lots of friends and a kind word for everyone. She never played favorites. She was a wonderful mother.

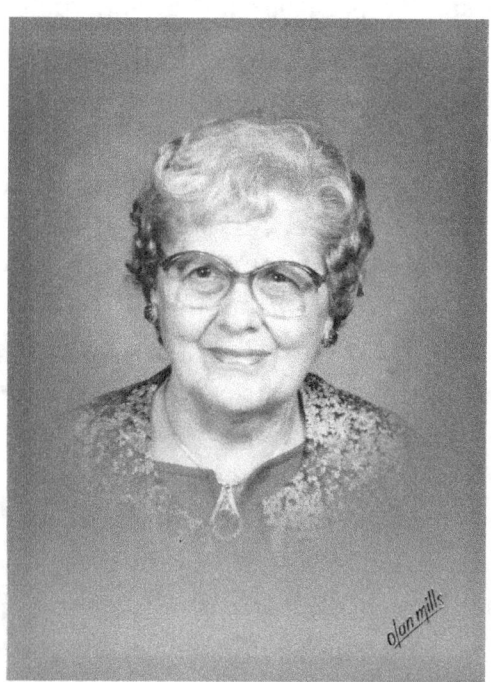

"Lottie"

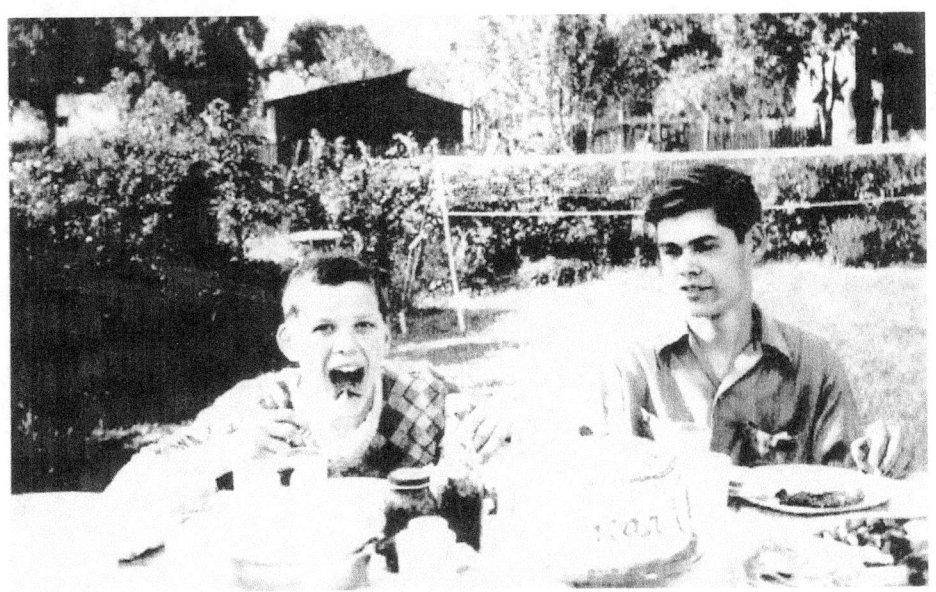

With Dean at 4th of July party at Helms'

CHAPTER 15
Playing the Uke

I probably was not what you would call a nerd in today's vernacular, but I was not very outgoing either and was fond of mathematics. I was more of a student than an athlete in school, and I guess that my desire to get good grades in school was based on my perceived need to satisfy the desires of my father. He always stressed the importance of doing the best that you could with the talents that you had, and that included doing the best that you could in school. So I was more the student than the socialite.

Around the time that I was in junior high, for some reason I started playing the ukulele. Since I had a pretty good voice, could carry a tune and could memorize music, I combined those talents and played a large variety of songs. Most were the old standards of the day.

One of my favorites on the uke was "Ain't She Sweet," and I could finger the tune on the keyboard. So over time, playing and singing became one of my primary social outlets. Throughout high school, I used the uke as my "alter ego" at parties and other social settings when I was too modest to use other techniques. That carried forth to college and beyond as well.

While a Supply Officer in the Navy, I commandeered a banjo that I could tune the same way as a ukulele, and I learned to play it pretty well. I had been sent by the commanding officer of our ship to a local supply depot in Norfolk, Virginia, to see if I could drum up anything to be used at a party we had scheduled for the ship's crew. The pickings were lean, and the only things that I could find that might be of any use were two banjos and a Chinese gong.

After some considered thought, I rejected the gong, but I signed the necessary paperwork, and showed up at the ship with two banjos. I am not sure to whom I gave the first banjo, but I took charge of the second. We didn't use the instruments at the ship's party but we kept them anyway. And after serving in the Navy, when folk singing became the rage, I learned Kingston Trio and other songs and was able to perform successfully at a number of folk events.

The banjo supplemented the uke and served me well when I was in the Jackson Ski club. It accompanied me to Pittsburgh, Princeton and Europe as well. Pat and I also learned to sing a couple of duets for parties. It is only recently, with the onset of peripheral neuropathy caused by an early chemo regimen, that the problems with my fingers have limited my playing. But the early start on the ukulele set me on a musical path that I have continued for more than fifty years. And I still can sing and do so in both the Voices Chorale and our Methodist Church choir.

CHAPTER 16
Dumb Things

I guess that everyone does some really dumb things in their life, things that you would like to take back if you had the chance. I know that I did. And one of the dumbest came the summer before I started college.

Bowling Green did not have a high school swim team. Maybe they do now, but they did not then. Since I pictured myself as a swimmer of sorts, I used to swim a lot to be ready in case I tried out for a swim team in college, little realizing that most college swimmers are probably on scholarship based on their records in high school. And that summer I decided that I would work on perfecting a racing dive.

So off I went to the community pool to practice racing dives. I did not have anyone to coach me. I just decided to start.

Well the first few practices went pretty well. I was getting a nice flat approach to the dive while working in the shallow end of the pool. But my next dive did not go so well. I hit the bottom of the pool. And when I shook myself off and checked myself off, I found out that I had chipped one of my top front teeth. Broke it right in half.

I went home to show my mother and she called our family dentist to set up an appointment. His advice was to wait until the nerves had a chance to withdraw from the edge of the tooth and then put on a cap. We asked how long you would have to wait and he recommended a couple of years. Now today you might not have to wait that long, but that was what he recommended with the dentistry that was practiced at that time. (And this was the same dentist that took out one of my wisdom teeth with a hammer and chisel.)

So I went off to college with one of my top front teeth broken in half. I didn't smile too much to hide my stupidity. And I had to bear with it for two years until I could get a cap put on that tooth that somewhat matched with the other front teeth.

I never did get on a college swim team. But if it was any consolation, during my senior year at Michigan, I was roommate to someone who was.

CHAPTER 17
The Suit

My father told me that in order to look good while he was teaching, he tried to buy a new suit and new pair of shoes every year. And he stressed quality. He said that you should spend the money to buy good quality clothes that will last and were worth the extra money. I discovered over time that, while working, it was a good idea. Dad did look pretty good when he got dressed up.

During my senior year at Bowling Green High School, I had competed in the tests for an NROTC (Naval Reserve Officer Training Corps) scholarship and was accepted. I had been eager to take the tests because a lot of it was math and that was my forte. It was also my way to avoid having to go to Bowling Green State University and end up being one of dad's business students, which was probably my Plan B.

In the NROTC, I could get to a nationally recognized school without costing my parents any money. It was called the Holloway Plan, named after the naval officer that created it and provided tuition, books and fees and $50 per month spending money to go to the school that accepted you.

I had listed a number of schools that I would have preferred, but I learned that the school where I was accepted in the program was the University of Missouri, a school that I knew little about. Because I was pretty much getting a "free ride," I accepted and prepared to go to start my freshman year. By the way, Carl Helms, and two of my other classmates were accepted in the program as well, at different schools. So Bowling Green High School had a pretty fair representation in the NROTC that year.

One of the things that I needed to take care of before going off to Columbia, Missouri, was my wardrobe. I did not have many clothes, and a lot of what I had were hand me downs from my older brother, Dean. That was the way the Cooke family worked. I am not sure how many of the clothes that Al, Dan and Jim had that were hand-me-downs, but I am sure that it was a significant amount.

Probably most of the money that my Mom spent raising the family went for food. She made sure that she took care of our needs. But we had to look after our wants. None of us had many clothes. But I had my money saved up from working at Kroger. So when I asked my dad what he recommended I spend my money on for college, he said that the first thing that I needed was a good suit. It sounded like a good idea.

Dad and I went down to his clothing store, Max Leitman's (he probably went there no more than once a year) and he told Max that we wanted to pick out a suit for his son. I believe, by the way, that it was the first time that I had been in the store, although I had passed by it many times on Main Street of Bowling Green. Well, they picked out this nice grey two-piece suit, double-breasted. I tried it on, got fitted and paid for it myself- $65 out of my college fund from my savings. Along with it a nice loud flowered tie to match, typical of the '50s.

Well, much to my surprise when I got to the University of Missouri, I found that the primary men's social attire was a blue blazer and grey slacks with a striped regimental tie. There was rarely a two-piece suit to be found, let alone a double-breasted. And no flowered ties. Any suits you saw were summer seersucker, which went at the local men's store for $25. So guess what. The nice high-priced suit that I had bought went into the closet. I may have worn it only once or twice. And if I needed something to wear, most of the time I would borrow a sport coat from one of my friends.

And oh yes, I did make friends. When the first semester grades came out and I had achieved four A's and a B+, I found I had a lot of friends, including fraternity members who were interested in having me pledge their fraternity in the spring pledge class. They were not interested at all in my suit; they were interested in my grades.

My first semester in college was quite a learning experience, socially as well as academically but I had learned that if I applied myself, I could compete at the college level.

CHAPTER 18
The Toledo Zoo/First Airplane Ride

Bowling Green, Ohio is about 24 miles south of Toledo. There were some attractions in Toledo that we would go to on occasion: the Toledo Mud Hens baseball team, the minor league affiliate of the Detroit Tigers; the Toledo Art Museum, a world class facility where I remember the treasures of the Berlin Art Museum making an appearance after the war; the race track where the Urschel boys and the Cooke boys would infrequently go to check out the horses when Hal was old enough to drive; and the Toledo Zoo, where our family would go and the school would also go for field trips. And guess what, our high school graduation class trip went to the Toledo Zoo. While other high schools were making trips to Washington and such places, we were getting on a bus and going to the Toledo Zoo. Big deal.

I am getting a bit ahead of myself, but when Pat, the children and I were living in Hong Kong in the mid-'80s, the Hong Kong International School, where Scott and Kelly went and graduated, had a spring program called "interim" where the students would go to some exotic place (at parent expense) and write up a report for credit. Our children went on such trips, as skiing in Japan, searching for the one-horned Rhino in Nepal, and living on a river boat in Kashmir, India. Not bad duty, but someone had to do it. So I had to frequently remind them that while they were traveling the world to write a school paper, there were people in the world who were driving

24 miles to go to the Toledo Zoo. So they should learn to appreciate what they have.

————————————

It was June 1953, the summer between my sophomore and junior years in college, when our high school graduating class had a reunion at the local community park, and I had my first airplane ride. One of our classmates, Bob Dimick, had received his pilot's license and was training in a plane at the local airport. Just days before our reunion, a tornado had struck Wood County, Ohio, and moved on up to Flint, Michigan where it did some serious damage. Bob asked some of us if we would like to take a plane ride to inspect the tornado damage, and I volunteered.

Well, the ride was awesome! Not just because it was my first ride in a plane, but because of what we saw flying over the area. You could see where the tornado had dropped down and taken out a barn, house or bridge, then risen up to cross a field and spared a structure and then dropped down somewhere else to do significant damage. Some places were destroyed and, just by chance, some places were spared. It was tremendous evidence of the force of nature as well as the coincidence of luck. After college, Bob joined the Air Force and, unfortunately, not long after, was killed in a plane crash in the line of duty.

But the ride did spark my adventuresome and travel spirits to seek out more opportunities for the same.

CHAPTER 19
"I'll Ne'er Forget My College Days"

(One of the University of Michigan college songs that we sang at most Glee Club concerts)

I am not sure what it is today, but when I started at the University of Missouri, I found out that it was primarily a social school with a fraternity and sorority system that was heavily based on legacies. If your father or mother had belonged to a particular fraternity or sorority at Missouri, the odds were that you were a shoo-in to get accepted to the same one. In fact, the week before school orientation was "Greek Week" and all of the potential pledges were invited up to meet with the various fraternities and sororities to make their choices.

The fraternities would have pretty much decided how many new pledges they wanted that year, and they would have identified the candidates from the incoming freshman class based on the recommendations of the parents and the fraternity alumni from around the state. Filling out the pledge class was pretty much a done deal, and you had to be pretty special to break the cycle. I learned that most of the out-of-state students at the school came for the School of Journalism and its daily newspaper. Very few were liberal arts or math majors, like me.

So while there were active dormitories at the University, most of the social life at the school revolved around the fraternity/sorority system. Many of the dorm residents were in the School of Agriculture and didn't care anyway. I arrived at the school during orientation week, which was the week after Greek Week so I didn't know what it was all about and at that time probably didn't much care.

My father had told me to focus on my studies and to set aside time each day to study my most difficult subjects. French Grammar was the most difficult one of my fall semester and I set aside two hours per day for that. The math subjects were easier than what I had studied in high school, so I breezed through those and then provided whatever extra time I had to the others. I had a pretty good fall semester grade-wise, with a 3.83 average. The only B was a B+ in my advanced English class where the Professor did not give any A's. (My Bowling Green High School background and my father's advice had put me in good stead.)

My grades caught the attention of the fraternity members in my classes and two fraternities, Phi Delta Theta and Phi Kappa Psi, made strong cases to me for my pledging their houses. I had several good friends in both fraternities and after deliberation I made my choice and pledged Phi Delt in their spring pledge class.

Now don't get me wrong. I was not just a student; I was also a singer and bridge player. I took a choral music class for credit, sang my first "Messiah" and also played a lot of bridge at the student union where I gained a reputation as a "country fair" player. Little did I know at the time that the bridge playing would hold me in good stead at the Phi Delt fraternity house.

Joining the fraternity turned out to be a good thing for me. It helped me get out of my shell and develop an ability to relate better to people. I did have to undergo an "interesting" pledge week to make the grade, including measuring fish lengths from one of the local drinking holes across town back to the fraternity house. One pledge held the clip board and pen and the other held the fish and the chalk. You would flip the fish lengthwise and mark with the chalk the length and the other pledge would count the number of fish-lengths on the clipboard. One "active" was standing by to make sure that we did not cheat. Every block or so, we would switch places for variety. It was a long night and a lot of fish lengths. There were several other equally "interesting" events that we had to endure over the week.

Also during pledge week we had to memorize the Greek alphabet, and rattle it off when asked by one of the actives. It is one of the things that I have never forgotten and I could probably rattle it off as fast now as I could then. It also often helps to know the Greek alphabet when doing crossword puzzles. They might ask you some trick question like what word in the Greek alphabet comes after zeta. If you had not been required to memorize the alphabet, you would not have a clue that the word is eta, followed by theta. Probably makes sense to the Greeks but not to me.

———————

We had a house mother named Mrs. Henderson, who liked to play bridge. If there were social nights when she did not have a partner, I frequently filled that role. It was at those times that the other brothers found out that I was a pretty good player.

In the basement of the fraternity house there was a room where we held chapter meetings, and I found out that further behind that room was a smaller room where the upper-class "brothers" held their card games. The "inner sanctum," so to speak. I knew that I was accepted when I was invited to play bridge with them there when I was just a sophomore. Private room with cigars and smoke, although I did not smoke at the time and found it a bit distracting.

One of the upperclassmen, Jack Revare, asked if I would be his partner in the University duplicate bridge competition. We ended up placing second place in the competition. The winners were a couple of grad students, so we considered ourselves the winners of the undergrad competition.

I could not match the brothers in clothes and social graces, but I did hold my own in grades and bridge playing.   I guess that evened things out.

CHAPTER 20
Summer NROTC Cruises

Naval Reserve Officer Training Corps (NROTC) students in the '50s were required to go on summer cruises of about six weeks in length. The cruises between the freshman and sophomore and the junior and senior years focused on the Fleet Navy of the high seas, while the NROTC program between the sophomore and junior years focused on Naval Air and the Marine Corps programs at locations in the US.

And so it was that the summer between my freshman and sophomore years at the University of Missouri found me in Norfolk, Virginia, ready to board the USS Missouri (BB-63), at that time one of the four battleships of the US Fleet. Our summer was to take us to Bergen, Norway, then to Portsmouth, England, and then back to the Naval Base at Guantanamo Bay, Cuba, for gunnery exercises, which included the firing of the 16-inch guns, the largest guns in the US military arsenal. It was to be my first time outside of the United States.

I don't remember a lot about the trip across the Atlantic, which took us about a week. We learned about life at sea, including the watch bill, swabbing the decks and becoming acquainted with the various departments of the ship. Watches were basically every four hours starting the day with the mid-watch of 0000 to 0400 (or midnight to 4 AM for those not familiar with military time) then continuing with the 0400 to 0800 watch, and so forth throughout the day for a total of six separate times. We frequently split the 1600 to 2000 watch in two, which gave both the 1600 to 1800 and the 1800 to 2000 groups a chance to eat dinner and rotated the watch assignments each day so you did not always have the mid-watch. (The ship's regular crew had the same watch assignment for a month.) We would vary our watch assignments by department, so we got a chance to stand watch in the gunnery department, the engineering department, the deck department, etcetera.

Then one morning we saw the fjords of Norway. We sailed up one of those and arrived at the charming city of Bergen, nestled in the base of a beautiful fjord. We anchored in the bay and those of us on liberty took the small boats to the fleet landing. Many of my shipmates immediately took off for the various bars that were located in the vicinity of the fleet landing. I was not into drinking beer at the time, so I remember taking long walks up in the hills surrounding the city and taking pictures of the ship resting in the harbor. Bergen was a fairly restful cruise destination, since there were not any side-trips available to provide any diversions. And my slide pictures are now occupying space in a slide tray in my basement.

Portsmouth, England, was a different story. Many of us took the side-trip to London; others took trips to other spots in the English countryside. I went to London; my first trip there of what would be many. I don't remember how many days we were in London but it was long enough to catch the changing of the guard, visit Parliament, Westminster Abbey, Tower Bridge, etcetera and catch a play. I believe it was the first time that I had ever seen a professional play. It was "The Boy Friend" with Julie Andrews in which she would later star on Broadway and which I would perform in myself when we lived in Pittsburgh. I also remember the drabness of the English food, mostly the beef with boiled potatoes and peas. There were probably other choices, but that is what I remember. Over the years, though, I believe that the food there has improved.

Guantanamo Bay, Cuba was a large Naval Base set on the eastern end of Cuba. It had a full range of Navy functions including a large Supply Base for replenishing the incoming ships. There was room in the harbor for the largest ships to anchor out in the bay while the smaller ships were able to tie up at the docks. For our shore leave you had to use the ship's small boat to get to and from the fleet landing at the base.

The primary purpose for going to Gitmo was to fire the 16-inch guns. There was an island located a little way from the base that was used for artillery practice. Firing the big guns was a big deal. There were not many places that the Navy could fire the guns. From the watches that we had stood at sea in the gunnery department, we knew how the guns were loaded and fired. We had also worked extensively with the 5-inch guns and had experience in aiming, loading, and firing those guns.

But the 16-inch guns were a special case. There were three gun turrets on the ship, two forward and one aft. When they were going to fire the guns, they would normally be rotated 90 degrees to one side to help absorb the blast. The ship would be at "general quarters" and announcements would be made when the guns were being loaded and when they were about to fire.

The noise that they made was tremendous. You were supposed to cover your ears during firing. I think that I did every time, but in recent years doctors have attributed some of my high frequency hearing loss to the effects of those big guns. I don't know if we ever hit any of the targets, but I do know that we made a lot of noise.

CHAPTER 21
The Marines Have Landed

Between the sophomore and junior years, NROTC students are assigned to Naval Air and Marine Corps training. For the Naval Air segment we went to the Naval Air Station at Cabaniss Field in Corpus Christi, Texas, where we went to mini flight school and participated in two flights in AT-6 two-seater prop trainers and one in a PBY flying boat. I was serving as one of the officers of the University of Missouri unit and was really embarrassed when I got sick during my first flight and threw up all over the cockpit of the plane.

I remember that they had a rule that if you got sick you had to clean up your own mess, but I was so sick that they laid me out on a table to recover and someone else, I don't know who, got the clean-up job. The pilot later came over and told me that it was not my fault since he thought that I was doing so well that he and another one of the pilots engaged in a little pseudo air battle at my expense.

I also got my first crack at a swimming race. For a diversion between our military activities, it was decided to have a swimming competition between some of the different schools. I decided to take a chance at the butterfly breast stroke, a stroke that I had been working on, but had never competed in. There were six of us in the race, two each from three different schools. The schools represented were mostly ones from the western part of the US that had NROTC programs; including Oklahoma, Stanford, Arizona, Colorado, etcetera. Some big hitters.

I don't remember who the other person was who competed for Missouri, but I assume that each of the other five were accomplished swimmers from college swim teams. The race was two widths of a large pool. Needless to say I ended up dead last. The other five were all very close to each other at the finish line. I was a half of the pool width behind. Not a sterling performance to say the least. And not one of which I am very proud. But I did fulfill my desire to compete in a NCAA type swimming competition.

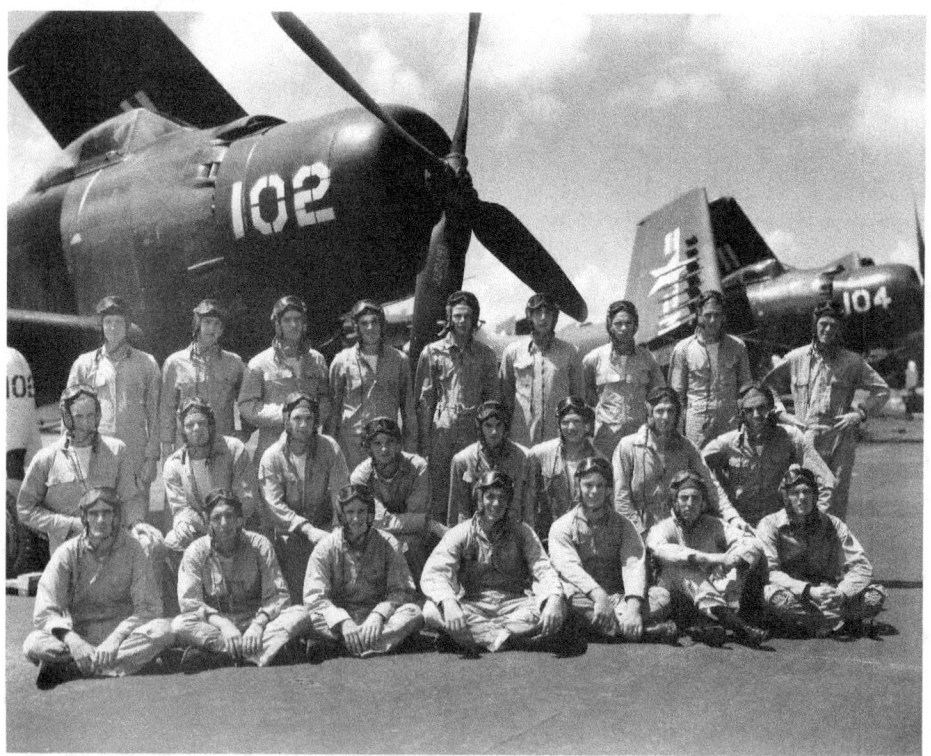

University of Missouri NROTC Unit at Corpus Christi, TX

We then took a flight in a personnel-equipped cargo plane to Little Creek, Virginia, home to some of the military's finest, the Marines.

We spent a couple of weeks living in Marine barracks, undergoing amphibious training and running obstacle courses at 0530 in the morning to toughen us up. To this day I don't know how I managed the Marine Corps obstacle courses but somehow I did. Maybe they had set up an easier course for the NROTC students.

After two weeks of training, we left the barracks and went to an APA personnel carrier ship right out of World War II. The bunks must have been stacked about eleven high. You would not want to have been in one of the top bunks and been a sleep walker or possibly have to go to the toilet. I was fortunate to have been in about the third tier.

After a day or two at sea, we were told to load up. We put on our landing gear and went to the side of the ship where they had rope ladders going down to the LCVP boats. LCVP stands for Landing Craft Vehicle Personnel and they are right out of the Normandy beaches in "The Longest Day."

We climbed down into our assigned craft and starting the circular staging activities. This is where the boats move into a circle until all of the boats are ready, and then they form a line abreast as they move toward shore. I don't remember how many of us were in each boat or how many boats were in each circle, but if you have ever seen any war movies of amphibious landings, you know what I am talking about.

At the signal, the boats all moved into a line abreast and headed for shore at Little Creek, Virginia which is a bit north of Virginia Beach. On the shore they had the reviewing force of Marine Corps officers: our instructors and their seniors sitting in football type bleachers to see how their charges of the previous two and one half weeks were going to perform.

We headed toward shore and at the proper time, the front gates of the boats were dropped and we attacked. Well, not exactly. We did not have guns ablaze as they did in the war movies, but we did have to jump into the water and got a little a wet as we made our way ashore. It was actually a great experience and gave us a much better appreciation as to what the troops went through on Omaha Beach or Guadalcanal.

I think that my development of a positive attitude may have started with my father, but my experience with the Marine Corps training at Little Creek certainly helped it along. I decided, however, at the end of the six-week program that I was going to stick to the Navy and bypass the Naval Air or the Marine Corps programs. In fact, I had already decided that I was going to transfer to the School of Business Administration at the University of Michigan and shift to the NROTC Naval Supply Corps program there.

CHAPTER 22
Summer NROTC Cruises-Part 2

The cruise in the summer between my junior and senior years was similar in that I was again on a battleship, but this time it was the USS Wisconsin (BB-64) and the cruise destinations were Glasgow, Scotland, and Brest, France, and then back to Gitmo. The side-trips were primarily to Edinburgh, Scotland, and Paris, France.

I took the side-trip to Edinburgh, and remember well Princes Street and the gardens where I would be singing with the University of Michigan Men's Glee Club five years later. I bought a sweater at one of the shops along Princes Street and have it to this day, although it is a little worn and I have had to have patches put along the sleeves. Overlooking Edinburgh is the famous Castle, which sits on a hill above the scene. It is a very interesting and enjoyable city, although I can't say too much for the weather.

From Brest, France, many of us took the long train trip to Paris. I remember that we stayed in a small hotel near the Arc de Triomphe, and we went all over the city. I can remember walking through Les Halles, the market area, when it came alive with vendors one morning about 4AM, and then walking back to the hotel. In the ensuing years, the market area there has been replaced by the Modern Art Museum. Paris, for midshipmen, was an exciting place. We went to the museums, the Tour Eiffel, and Notre Dame, but we also went to see some of the shows such as the Moulin

Rouge and the Follies Bergere. I believe all of us had a good time, and little did I know, at the time, that 25 years later, I would be living in Paris with IBM.

After returning to Brest, we had time for one more tour to the westernmost point of France on the tip of the Ocean where you could experience the full force of the Atlantic waters. Then we made the trip back to Gitmo for R & R and the firing of the 16-inch guns.

One variation on this trip was a relationship that I had struck up at the University of Michigan with a tenor member of the Glee Club who was also in the NROTC, Bob Ely. He and I had started singing duets during our college days, and would often double date and entertain our dates with some of our songs.

We worked up a program of songs on the ship and auditioned for the show that was to be held on the fantail to entertain the crew during our trip from France to Gitmo. We were selected for the program and also for another performance that was held in the officers' wardroom.

We called ourselves "The Admirals Waiters" and wore Scottish tams that we had purchased in Glasgow, actual waiters jackets borrowed from the Captain's wardroom and swimming trunks. Songs included "Down by the Riverside," "Persian Kitten," "George Jones," and the Bing Crosby and son hit song, "Play a Simple Melody." I normally sang the melody and Bob would add a tenor line about a third higher. If I say so myself, we were a bit of a hit!

The USS Wisconsin ship's newspaper had the following to say in its 1 September 1954 issue-"Bing and Gary Crosby couldn't have far surpassed the singing duo of midshipman 1/c Ely and Cooke- the "Admiral's Waiters." Their voices matched as well as their costumes and the entertainment they provided was top drawer."

Bob and I went on to have leads in the following next year's production of the "Michigan Union Opera" in Ann Arbor, and on the road tour in New York between Christmas and New Years. We also performed in music activities at the Naval Supply Corps School in Athens, Georgia, the following summer.

Several years ago my wife, Pat, and I vacationed at Virginia Beach and we went to Norfolk where the USS Wisconsin is permanently tied up as a museum. It was my first visit to the ship since the cruise of 1954 and it was a nostalgic experience to stand on the fan-tail of the ship where Bob and I had performed so many years previously. It was a pleasant reminder of the days when I was making maximum use of my musical skills.

It was after my junior cruise that I decided to hitchhike home, taking in a couple of locations that I had wanted to see. I had already experienced hitchhiking from Bowling Green to and from Ann Arbor during my Junior year without any problems. I had a sign with "Ann Arbor" on one side and "Bowling Green" on the other that I used to go back and forth to school. It worked just fine and I rarely waited any length of time to get a ride.

I had spent some time after an earlier cruise visiting with a University of Missouri friend in Williamsburg, Virginia and after that stay I had taken the train home. But this time I wanted to see Gettysburg, Pennsylvania, and Niagara Falls and that would require some travel by car, therefore hitchhiking was the answer.

I had found out that if I wore my NROTC uniform and stood by the side of the road, it was not long before I had a ride. I don't remember how many rides that it took, but I made it to both of my primary destinations. I do remember that the most difficult leg of the trip was from Niagara Falls to Detroit, going across Canada.

Hitchhiking was relatively safe in those days, or so I thought, but I would not recommend it at all today. It would be too dangerous with all of the kooks on the road. But it was an extension of my love of travel.

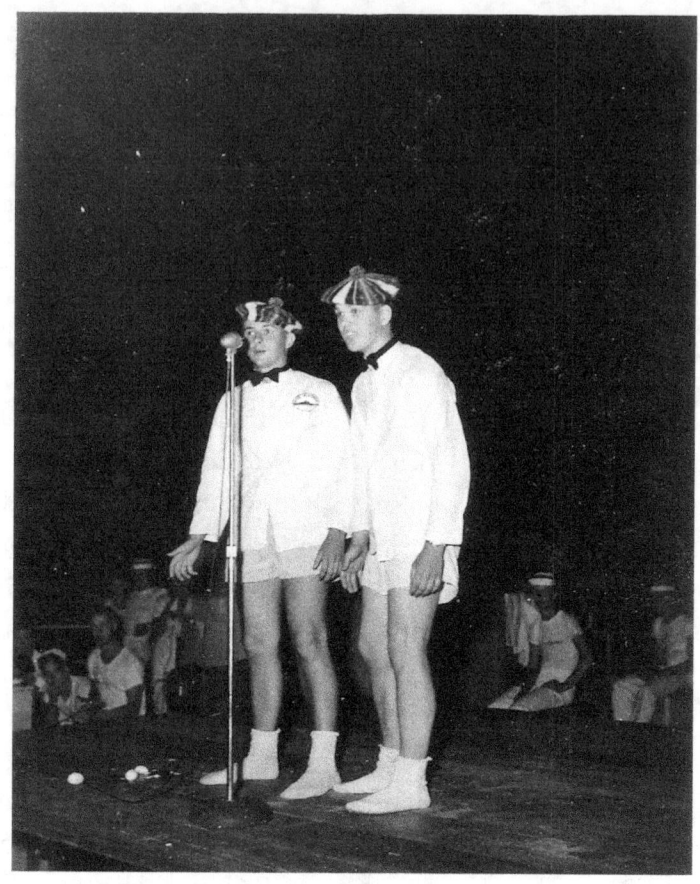

"The Admiral's Waiters"-1954

CHAPTER 23
I'll Ne'er Forget My College Days, Part 2

In the fall of 1953, I started my junior year at the University of Michigan. It was a much different school than the University of Missouri, where I had spent my first two years. More focus was on scholastic achievement and less on social graces. However, at the Michigan Alpha chapter of Phi Delta Theta, where I was a transfer student, more focus was on athletic achievement. We were probably known as a jock house, although there were a variety of skills in the membership. And as I have previously identified, I was anything but a jock.

But I did find a group of guys in the fraternity house that liked to sing, and in the fall of my junior year I joined several of them in auditioning for the University of Michigan Men's Glee Club. A couple of the other brothers and I made the cut and for the next two years, the glee club became one of my major school activities.

We sang in white tie and tails and were considered one of the top men's glee clubs in the country. We did a couple of tours a year around the US and cut a couple of records. It was a lot of fun, and I rejoined the group after I returned to graduate school following my three year-stint in the Navy. It was a further development of my musical skills.

My roommates at the Phi Delt fraternity house in my senior year, Tim Reiman and Bill McArthur, were both in the ROTC, one in the Army and the other in the Air Force. They were both in Scabbards and Blades, the ROTC honorary society. Imagine my surprise one night in the spring of my senior year when I was awakened during the night to find both of them at the foot of my bed, in full uniforms, to roust me out to be initiated into the honorary.

I continued to get good grades at Michigan, got a job offer from General Electric for their management training program, graduated with distinction (was selected for Beta Gamma Sigma, the business school Phi Beta Kappa) and immediately after graduation in June 1955 was commissioned in the Navy as an Ensign in the Naval Supply Corps.

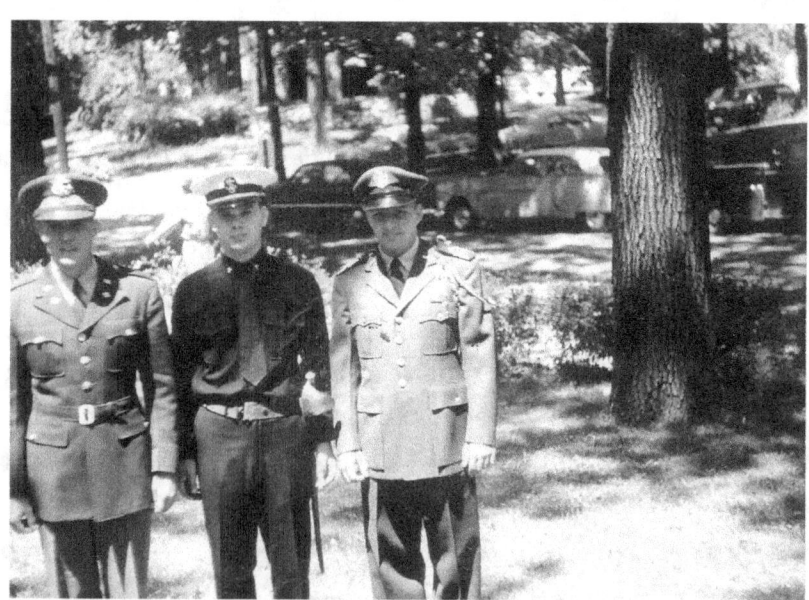

With Tim Reiman and Bill McArthur at Ann Arbor

CHAPTER 24
The Sixth Fleet

As a newly minted Supply Corps Ensign, I was required to spend my first summer after commissioning at the Naval Supply Corps School in Athens, Georgia, with students from all of the other universities that had Supply Corps NROTC training. Two of the other schools represented were Princeton, where I would later live, and Miami of Ohio, which my brother, Dan would later attend.

There I learned all of the tools of the trade of a supply officer, with a primary focus on the disbursing function. After completing the school, in September 1955, I was assigned to the heavy cruiser, the USS Albany, CA123, as Disbursing Officer. It was stationed at the Naval Piers in Norfolk, Virginia and soon after I arrived at the ship in the fall of 1955, we went on a shakedown cruise in the Caribbean to San Juan, Puerto Rico, to orient the new crew.

I found out that one of the officers in the Gunnery Department, Pete Appeddu, was also a University of Michigan grad and lived in Perrysburg, Ohio, about 20 miles north of Bowling Green. He had been a year ahead of me at school and I had not known him before. But it was convenient to have him live close by. He had a car and we made the trip back to Ohio together during home leave that Christmas.

In January 1956 we were due to depart for six months as part of the Sixth Fleet, the fleet assigned to the Mediterranean area. Pete wanted to leave his car at home during that cruise so we needed to fly back to Norfolk after the home leave and joined up at the Toledo Airport for the flight back. It was my first commercial airline flight, on a prop plane called the Lockheed Constellation. That is about all I remember about it so it must have been uneventful.

But the subsequent trip across the Atlantic was anything but uneventful. We encountered one of the worst storms in memory for many of the crew. There were two heavy cruisers going over together, the Albany and the Newport News. And we rocked from side to side and took heavy waves. We tilted so far that the water was coming up over the lifeboats. I believe that there was some talk of turning around but that was not done. There was a lot of damage to both of the ships.

And talk about being sea sick! There were only a few of the most experienced crew who were not affected. After about four days of this, things finally settled down and we made a non-scheduled stop in Gibraltar, where both ships were put into dry-dock for emergency repairs. We got a chance to tour the port and see the famous apes on the "Rock."

You would think that I would have learned my lesson about buying clothes, but a number of my fellow officers were taken with the Gibraltar tailor shops where you could buy Harris Tweed sport coats and tailored suits and so forth at a good price. Well, I went shopping with some of them one day and did end up with a sport coat and a new grey suit (to be fitted). But before the fittings on the suit were complete, we learned that the repairs on the ships were complete and we were going to set sail for our next port (Naples). I had to get busy to fill up one of my safes with a supply of foreign currency for all of the ports that we were going to visit in France, Italy, Greece, Lebanon and Spain. We also learned that we would have to pre-pay for the clothes and they would be sent to us via some other Navy ship that was going to meet up with us later in the Med.

When we got to Naples, many of the officers made a side trip to Rome wearing Gibraltar sport coats. The fit of the my sport coat was not so bad, although those of us that bought the Harris Tweed learned first-hand that it is a heavy fabric and not too well suited for the Mediterranean weather. When the grey suit arrived, not only did it not fit right, but it had been cut a bit extreme for my taste and I don't believe that I ever wore it. If memory serves me, I gave it away to a charity when we returned to home port in Norfolk. At least at that time I was making a bit more money so the loss did not hit my pocket book as badly as the double-breasted experience at Missouri.

There was not much military excitement going on in the Med at that time, so we started a process of about a week at sea followed by about a similar time in a port of call. There were some interesting experiences, including afternoon gin and tonics with the officers on the deck of a British man-of-war. From Naples, we went to Genoa, Italy; Cannes, France; and Athens, Greece. Next stop was Beirut, Lebanon.

It was while we were in Greece, that I received my orders to take over as Supply Officer on the USS Leary, DDR 879. This was called independent duty and was a step up from the job that I had on the Albany. We discovered that the Leary was due in Beirut several days after the Albany was due to leave there, so it was decided to offload me in Beirut on another US ship until the Leary arrived.

The Albany left Beirut with the Marine guard in full regalia, flags flying and the ship's band playing. It was several hours before the ship that I was being temporarily transferred to was due to arrive, and I was left on the dock in my dress uniform with the sea chest that the Albany's carpenters had made for me, awaiting the ships arrival. I was amidst a large number of swarthy dock workers, wondering if I had made the right decision. I was the only American-looking face in sight. In today's world, one never would have done it. Finally after several hours of anxious waiting, I saw a group of destroyers coming into view and the ship finally arrived. I don't remember its name but I was really glad to see it.

I had several days on my hands with no assigned duties to perform until the Leary arrived. Three of the officers on this destroyer decided to join me and hire a cab to go to Baalbek, an ancient Roman town located several hours outside of Beirut through the Biblical valley of "milk and honey." We made the trip to the ancient town where there were a number of archeological studies going on among the ruins. It had a well-preserved number of ruins and was quite a site. One ruin was called the Temple of Bacchus and was dedicated to the love of wine. Having already seen the coliseum of Rome and the acropolis of Athens, I got yet another view of the history of mankind, an interest I still have to this day. I was also getting a full dose of international travel to satisfy that urge as well.

CHAPTER 25
The Bos and the Fongs

In the Navy, I had home leave twice a year. I tried to get home for Christmas and then for a week during the summer. It was during a summer leave that I first encountered the Bos. My sister, Janet, was dating a Bowling Green State University basketball player named Tom Benbrook, and he was spending a bit of time at our house getting into the good graces of my younger brothers, Al, Dan and Jim, while romancing my sister.

Tom had good naturedly started calling them Al-bo, Dan-bo, and Jim-bo and that was the accepted practice when I showed up on home leave. Well for some reason, I questioned the naming practice and wondered why they could not be called by other names such as Al-Fong and Dan-Fong. I believe that we had a Chinese college or exchange student living in the basement room in our home at that time and perhaps that is where I got the idea. In any case, we now had two naming conventions and they stuck.

For many years afterwards we have encountered situations where the family is divided into two groups, such as for charades, or other team events. And several of our nieces and nephews got into the act and with relish, divided the teams into the Bos and the Fongs. So the practice that got started sometime in the late '50s has survived for over fifty years. Even now at family reunions or dinners we may find nametags labeled with a Bo or a Fong. I don't think that many of the family members have a clue as to how the names got started, and may not know who is a Bo and who is a Fong, but it is just one of those family things that just lingers on. It is clear that I am in the Fong ranks. One of my brothers just calls me Fong.

CHAPTER 26
Schuster

When I first joined the USS Leary, DDR 879, the radar picket destroyer where I spent twenty six months as Supply Officer, one of the first people that I met was Schuster, my First Class Supply Clerk. I never knew his first name. To me he was just Schuster. He was an expert in everything related to the supply department; the disbursing function (although I did have a talented disbursing clerk and was fairly self-sufficient in that role myself), the storekeeping function, the ships store, and even the commissary and the laundry. For a new untested Ensign Supply officer, he was a godsend. He was familiar with all of the reports that had to be written and submitted and was just a valuable person to have around.

Schuster did have some faults. He kept a "Mediterranean" wife in Cannes, and he was pretty smug about all of the things that he knew. But given that my knowledge of many of the supply office functions came from the schoolbooks in Athens, Georgia, it was helpful to have someone around that knew the ropes and could help me in the learning process.

As I progressed in my knowledge of what I had to do as the officer in charge of the Supply Department on the ship, and went through a couple of the monthly reporting cycles, my level of competence increased and I used Schuster more as a sounding board and less as a crutch.

It was much to my surprise when, in the last week of our Mediterranean tour, I learned that Schuster had been written up for selling sea-store cigarettes over the side of the ship. The sea-store cigarettes were the ones that were tax free, and should only be sold at sea to members of the ship's crew. The going price for sea-store cigarettes at the time was $.08 a pack or $.80 a carton for regular cigarettes like Camels or Lucky Strike, and $.10 a pack or $1.00 a carton for Winston's or other longer brands. On shore the cigarettes would sell for many times their sea-store rate. Compare those prices to the prices of cigarettes today.

Schuster was caught illegally selling cases of cigarettes to foreign nationals who would come by the Leary at night in a small boat to make the exchange, trading money for cigarettes. What he was charging for a case and how much profit the nationals would make was not relevant. He was toast!

My days of relying on Schuster were over. Fortunately, I was pretty much prepared to go it alone. And when we returned to Norfolk, he was escorted off of the ship in disgrace and I was assigned a new 1st Class Storekeeper. I don't know whatever became of Schuster.

I learned that the one person I could trust all of the time was myself, so to the extent possible I had to know everything that there was to know about any job that I had. This forced me to develop planning/organizing skills a bit earlier than I might have planned on. And those skills have helped me up to the present day.

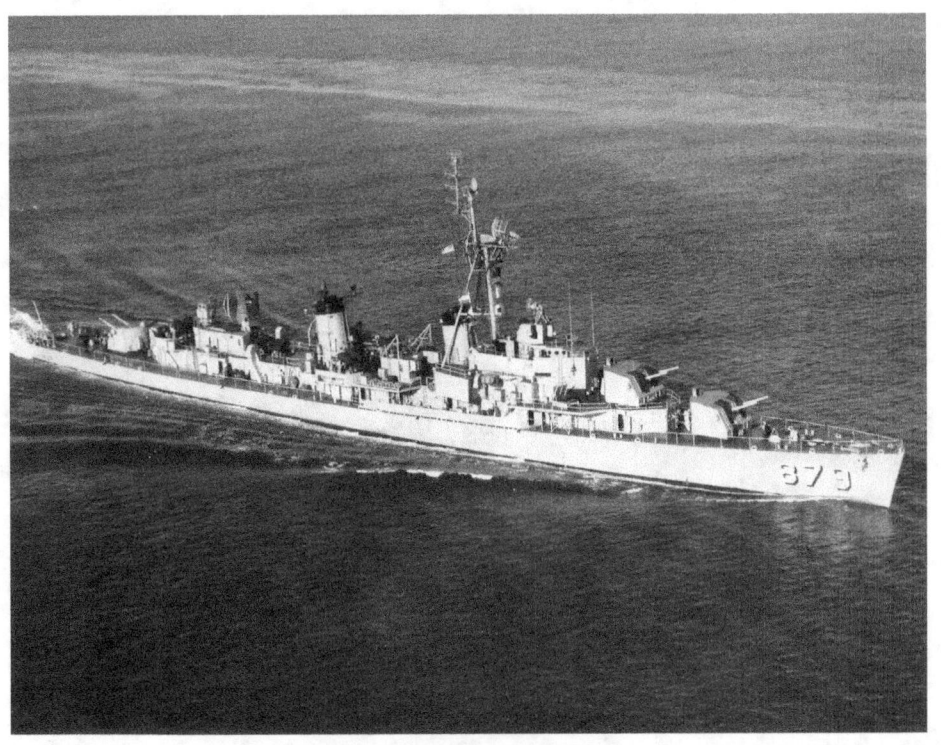

USS Leary (DDR-879)

CHAPTER 27
My First Car

The USS Leary tied up at the Destroyer/Submarine piers in Norfolk, which were several miles from where the larger ships like the USS Albany tied up. The Albany and the Leary were also on separate deployment schedules. So in making the change of ships, I had also lost my ride to and from Ohio with Pete Appeddu. This made it necessary for me to buy a car. Unlike the common practice today, I did not have a car of my own either in high school or college.

I had been the Boy Scout leader for a Cub Scout den in our neighborhood in Bowling Green, Ohio. The lady, who was the our den mother, told me that she had a car from one of her deceased relatives parked in a garage across the street from her house that she was interested in selling. So I went to take a look. It was a stick shift Chrysler without a radio and without air conditioning, but it ran well. And she was willing to sell it for, as I remember, $250. It had the initials LC on the side that stood for Loren Campbell, who had been the previous owner. Some people thought that the initials the stood for some member of the Cooke clan, but that was not so.

So I bought it. The trip back to Norfolk was a bit over 12 hours: six hours to the Breezewood exit on the Pennsylvania Turnpike, and six hours from there down Route 17 to Norfolk. In those days getting AC and a radio in a car were options and not standard. Driving back to Norfolk I found that if I kept the windows open, the lack of

AC was diminished, particularly in the hilly sections of the drive. And I developed a habit of singing to myself to offset the lack of a radio. It was not ideal but it worked.

I had that car until after I joined IBM.

CHAPTER 28
"Mister Roberts"

I enjoyed Henry Fonda in the movie "Mister Roberts." Toward the end of the movie there is a scene where he is on the supply ship heading away from the war. Looking out on the horizon he sees a large flotilla of war ships heading in the opposite direction toward the Japanese war zone. The sea is filled with ships of every description, battleships, cruisers, destroyers, aircraft carriers, support vessels, everything you can think of. All going to war and he is going the other way. You wonder how so many ships could have been mobilized in such a manner. Well, I have had a personal experience that reminded me of the movie.

It was the fall of 1956 and we were doing some maneuvers off of Norfolk with the other destroyers of our squadron when we got orders to proceed to port immediately to restock the ships. When we arrived back in Norfolk the orders for delivery of supplies had already been processed for the four destroyers in our squadron, the Leary, Steinaker, Vesole and Wood. We proceeded to load supplies and take on fuel round the clock. Something was up, but we did not know what it was. We took on replacements for our rocking-cradle radar and foul weather gear and everything else in between. I had never gone through such a supply replenishment process. After about three days of this we set sail for parts unknown.

We basically sailed due East but no one knew the final destination. Finally, after several days at sea, some secret orders came in and
at least the captain and the executive officer (second in command)
knew what was going on. I was one of the junior officers on board, so
I should have been one of the last to know, but I was also one of the officers trained in the crypto process and had a secret security clearance.

And then the morning arrived. I had gotten up early because I
had a sense that something was going on. And when I looked out
on the horizon, it was a sight for Mr. Roberts' eyes. There were more
ships than I had ever seen at one time. There must have been close
to 50 ships. Three aircraft carrier groups with their supporting ships.
Cruisers. At least 24 destroyers (three groups of eight each to support
each of the carriers), tankers, and supply ships. The sea was full, and
we were right in the middle of it.

And where were we? It turned out that we were off the coast of
Portugal at the entrance to the Mediterranean. One of the three carrier groups had just left duty in the sixth fleet. One of the groups had
just arrived from Norfolk as the replacement fleet, and one had been
sent over on special duty if needed. We were part of that last group.
The reason for all of this activity was the hubbub that was going on
with Israel, France, and Britain versus Egypt over the Suez Canal.
The US marines were on standby. It was a major international crisis.

After several days the crisis had abated and the three carrier
groups had separated: one to go back to the states, one to go into the
Mediterranean to take up duties in the sixth fleet, and us to sail off
the coast of Portugal in case we were needed. So that one morning
was the one time you were able to see such a fleet.

After about a week of sailing around, some higher-up determined
that we needed liberty and we landed in Lisbon for shore leave. We
stayed for a few days and then regrouped and sailed back to Norfolk
where we arrived in time for home leave over Christmas.

I never saw so many ships in one place at one time again.

CHAPTER 29
Little Creek Officers Club

The primary role of the USS Leary, DDR 879, was to plane-guard for aircraft carriers. This meant that we positioned ourselves off of the starboard stern of the carrier during flight operations to pick up any pilots that might have to "ditch" during carrier landings. Most of our operations were either off of our homeport of Norfolk or in the Caribbean, where the weather was more predictable.

If we were in port on a Thursday night, which was about twice a month, it was fun to go to the Little Creek Officers Club. Yes, this was the same Little Creek where I spent three weeks during my second midshipman summer. Well, on Thursday night they had a piano player at the club lounge and sold quarts of beer for a quarter. The piano player knew all of the old songs and it made for a very enjoyable evening, particularly if you had been out at sea for a couple of weeks.

They even published a songbook with all of their favorites. I found a copy in the basement of our house in some of my stuff. One of the favorites that I took up in my ukulele-banjo days was "Seven Old Ladies Locked in the Lavatory." It goes "Oh dear, what can the matter be. Seven old ladies locked in the lavatory" and so on through seven verses. A good party song.

I would assume that the same piano player is no longer there and beer is no longer a quarter, but I would hope that they have continued the singing tradition. Over the years it was a lot of fun and a good break from sea duty.

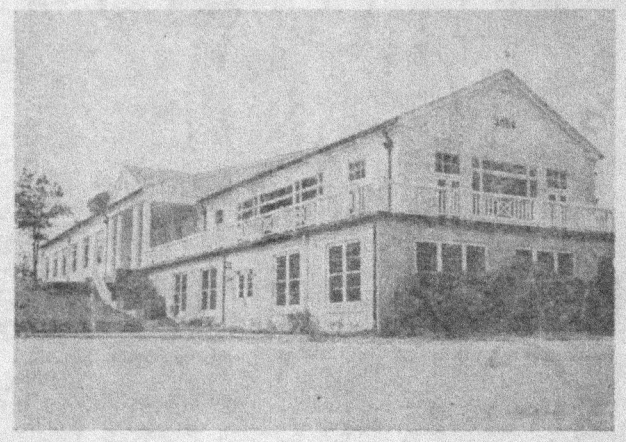

Little Creek, Virginia Officers Club Songbook

CHAPTER 30
Cartan Tours

Jim Shortt was the Glee Club Faculty Advisor of the Michigan Men's Glee Club during the time that I was in the club. He was also a good friend of mine and a good bridge player; we frequently played together. What I did not know about him when I was in school was that during the summer months, he worked for the Cartan Tour Company, a Chicago based tour operator that did high end tours. Many of the tours that Jim did were to Hawaii, and he would tell me about how he would host the cocktail parties for the guests at some lavish Oahu hotel while managing the tours.

During one of my home leaves before I left the Navy, he talked to me about how I might enjoy a summer job as a tour manager before going back for my MBA at Michigan. (I had pretty much decided that after leaving the Navy, the best thing for me would be to go back for an MBA to prepare to enter the job market, since the country was in a recession at the time.) .

He arranged for me to have an interview and so, off I went off to Chicago to interview for a job as a tour manager. I was accepted; not for the plush Hawaiian gig that Jim Shortt had described but for an entry level two week train tour of National Parks and the Colorado Rockies. An on-the-ground type of experience. And no drinking with the tourists.

And so it was that a couple of weeks after I left the service (I was not formally discharged until ten years later), I was in Chicago's Union Station getting my instructions from the local Cartan representative. I was given my transportation, meal and hotel vouchers, and contact instructions and sent on my way with about 30 travelers in tow. We caught the Sunday evening train from Chicago's Union Station to Three Forks, Montana.

We arrived in Three Forks mid-morning and were met by a tour bus that took us to Virginia City, Montana. There we had a chance to meander around the town, visit the "honky-tonk" sights and see the "melodrama" at the Silver Dollar Saloon. The next morning we were on our way to Yellowstone National Park where we stayed first at the Yellowstone Lodge for several days to see Old Faithful and the other sights there. We then went up to the Canyon Lodge, by the Grand Canyon of the Yellowstone which I previously did not even know existed.

The bus drivers on our tours were all well trained guides and would give the local tour information. During the early part of the tour, I would use the bus microphone to entertain the crowd by singing songs during the travel legs on the tour.

However, one of the boy travelers in my first tour group, age about ten, kept after me asking if this was my first time on this trip. I must have appeared somewhat nervous to him, although I thought I was carrying off my uncertainty pretty well. I did have a small bag that I carried all of my important documents in that I kept pretty close to me on the train. Maybe he sensed something from that. In any case, the bus drivers knew that there were some "green" tour managers that they had to contend with, and they tried to make it easy on us. It added an additional dimension to my first trip and I never did admit it to the boy that it was, indeed, my virgin trip.

Next, Yellowstone to the Grand Tetons. The Tetons were probably one of the most dramatic sites of the whole trip. We stayed at the Grand Teton Lodge with soaring picture-window views of the mountains. Truly awesome. I would have to say that with the Cartan tours you had nice digs and nice meals. (And I got to sign all of the checks.)

By now we were at the end of our first week, and we caught the Saturday night train to Salt Lake City to visit the Mormon Tabernacle in time for the Sunday morning service. (It was one of the featured spots on the tour, but out of my four tours that summer we only made it in time to hear the choir sing on two occasions.)

The bus then went on to the Great Salt Lake, not a very exciting experience. After my first trip to the Great Salt Lake, I opted to stay at the hotel during the rest of the trips, telling the tour group that I had to get caught up on my paperwork. And then I would spend a few hours at the hotel pool with a couple of the tour managers from other companies that I had crisscrossed with over the weeks.

From Salt Lake City we took the D&RGW train to Colorado: officially the Denver and Rio Grande Western, but known affectionately as the Degenerate and Rapidly Growing Worse. We traveled through the Great Gorge to Colorado Springs. This was one of those train trips that you read about, where you are in the observation car with breathtaking views out at the mountains and cuts through the deep passes and gorges as you rattle along the tracks. And they serve the most delicious rainbow trout in the dining car.

There was a girl with a guitar that got on the train in Salt Lake City and we passed some of the time singing folk songs

At Colorado Springs, we took the obligatory trip up Pike's Peak and stayed at the Broadmoor. We had nice rooms and very nice meals. Then on to Estes Park and the trip up the Trail Ridge Road over the top of Rocky Mountain National Park, down to Grand Lake and then back to Denver for a city tour and the train trip back to Chicago.

We saw a lot in two weeks. Had four night train rides, some excellent hotels, and some great meals. And after the first trip, I did not have to endure any more questioning ten year olds. I was the experienced expert. I did three more such trips over the course of the summer and became quite knowledgeable on the sites that we saw. And I got the chance to add a number of national parks to my travel resume.

CHAPTER 31
Thinking about a job with IBM

I think that my father had wanted me to get a job with IBM after I received my MBA from The University of Michigan. Several of his students had taken jobs with IBM, including one who worked in the nearby Toledo office, and he must have felt that I was just as competent as they were. When I arrived home from the Navy and in the time before and after the Cartan Tour experience, he would have this former student, and others, stop by the house to talk to me. He also arranged for me to meet with former students that worked at nearby corporations, such as Marathon Oil, in Findlay, Ohio where they were gaining experience with IBM computers. Dad must have realized then that computers were going to be a big wave in the future and that with my skill in math, it could be a good fit for me.

The former student from the IBM Toledo office was the one who talked to me the most. He told me about the experiences he had telling senior executives of his customers about computers. He knew more about computers than the execs did and that gave him a feeling of equality even though he was many years younger. He spoke to me about the training that he had and the spark that he gained out of making a sale. I told him that I was not sure that I wanted to be a salesman. He said that from the early sales training classes, which were excellent, there were other routes that you could take with IBM but that the sales training route was the best one for advancement.

I guess I was convinced. In high school, I had been a fan of Winston Churchill, possibly because his initials, WTC, and mine are the same. And IBM had an organization with the same initials, the World Trade Corporation, which handles all of its international activities. I thought it would be prophetic if I was hired by IBM and ended up in the World Trade organization. So when I left for Ann Arbor in the fall, I was hopeful that I could land a job with IBM and see where it took me. And early in the fall interview process, I was offered a job as a sales trainee in the IBM Dearborn office to start in June after graduation.

And my Dad was probably doubly proud when one of my younger brothers, Dan, after graduating from Miami University in Ohio four years later, landed a job with the IBM office in Cincinnati, Ohio.

In those days, IBM was a prestigious company and getting a job with IBM was considered to be a plum job. But times change and, while IBM has been through some difficult times in the past twenty years or so, lately it has been coming back strong in the software and services businesses.

CHAPTER 32
University of Michigan MBA

To be perfectly honest, I did not have a particularly difficult time in getting my MBA. My dad had mentioned that if I wanted to go to someplace else like Harvard, he had some contacts and would write me a recommendation. But I had taken advanced credit courses while an undergrad at Michigan and needed only 27 hours of course material to get an MBA there. So Michigan it was. My most difficult time was probably not with my courses but with my faculty advisor, who had his own ideas about the courses that I should be taking.

It was the start of the age of computers. The university had just procured an IBM 650 computer and was teaching courses on computer sciences and programming. There were also a growing number of related mathematical courses, and it was there that my advisor directed me. Because of my math background, he was convinced that I was a good candidate for the courses in matrix algebra and linear programming being taught in the mathematics department. I was not convinced that the courses were practical enough; that they were too theoretical. But my advisor prevailed. And so I went.

In the matrix algebra class I learned how to figure out the solution and then work backward to the proof, and in the other, it was one of those professors who wrote math on the blackboard with his right hand and erased it with his left; filling up blackboards along the way. Somehow I just figured that one out and got As in both courses along the way. However, I don't believe that I ever used any of the information that I learned in those two classes anytime in my 30-year IBM career.

The course that probably helped me the most in my career was the one on programming the IBM 650 computer. We used an assembly language called SOAP (Symbolic Optimal Assembly Program), would key our instructions out in punched cards, leave them to be processed overnight, and then stop by the computer lab the next morning to get the results. Knowing how to program probably gave me a leg up on the other IBM new hires.

My advanced Accounting courses were fairly straightforward. I actually adapted matrix algebra to one course, which pleased my advisor. The course that probably upset him the most was one that I enjoyed the most, Music Lit, where we studied the music of Mozart, Brahms, Beethoven, et al. This was one that I kind of snuck in on him.

It is that course that I remember well today and the one that taught me a love of classical music. We studied the sonata allegro, using the Mozart 40th symphony as the structure. And we spent an extra amount of time on Beethoven's 3rd symphony, the Eroica; and Brahms 1st. We also spent time with Handel, Haydn, Tchaikovsky, Franck, and others. No choral music, just symphonic. I picked up my love of classical choral music later.

So with 15 hours of course work in the fall and 12 in the spring, I earned my MBA. In the spring, I went to school only on Monday, Wednesday and Friday. On Tuesday and Thursday, I had interviewed for and landed a job working with the Internal Audit department of the University, auditing the cash funds of smaller organizations on the campus. I was one student out of about a dozen auditors. It was a good experience in real world work and I earned my spending money.

I did go to the graduation exercise to be awarded my diploma. A number of my classmates did not go and just went to the graduate office afterwards to get pick theirs up. But I was finally done with school and ready to go to work, after my next trip to Europe.

CHAPTER 33
Michigan Men's Glee Club

What I really enjoyed throughout my graduate year at the University of Michigan was singing with the Michigan Men's Glee Club. I had to audition again to gain admission, but that was not a problem, and so I was singing as a grad student with many of the same students that were freshman when I had first started in the club. That summer we were going on a European singing jaunt for a couple of months.

I still had my job offer from GE from undergrad days, but in the fall of graduate school, I had interviewed with IBM and was offered a job in sales training in the Dearborn office which I had accepted. They wanted me to start in June after I graduated, but with the summer tour coming up, I did not want to until September 1. I was very nervous about telling the branch manager that I would not be able to start until then, but he must have been eager to have me and did not bat an eye to tell me that September 1 was OK with him. So I made my plans to travel to Europe that summer with the Glee Club.

One of the highlights of the tour was the participation in the International Eisteddfod (Music festival) being held in Llangollen, Wales featuring male choruses from all over Europe.

We went to Europe on a student ship, The Seven Seas, out of Montreal. It was a somewhat rough trip, and our director Dr. Philip Duey was sick for much of the voyage, so our accompanist had to handle many of the rehearsals. But we enjoyed the trip. The Notre

Dame Glee Club was also on the boat as were a number of other students making the trip for the summer. One of the favorite pastimes was Bingo, played each night in the ship lounge.

We were due to arrive in Southampton, England, in time to catch a waiting bus to Llangollen, Wales, arriving there early in the evening where we were to meet families that were going to put us up for the night. But the ship was late. And the bus was late. And so we were late. Rather than arriving in Wales to meet our hosts in early evening, we arrived well after midnight when most of them had left the churchyard meeting area (it was the church at Chirk) and gone home.

So our tour organizer had to roust out the hosts and get us to bed, probably no earlier than 3 or 4 in the morning. But we were young and could get by without a lot of sleep. About 7 the next morning, we were all up and organized to get to the singing grounds for rehearsal for the competition.

We were singing three songs, two required numbers and one of national origin. I remember that the required songs were Confitemini Domino in Latin and El Grillo (The Cricket) in Italian. Our optional number was a number by an American composer called "Stomp your foot." We had practiced those numbers so much that I could probably sing them today with a limited amount of rehearsal. In any event, we were competing against some of the best male choruses in Wales, not to say some of the best in Europe. There were eighteen singing groups from ten countries in the competition. We were the only American group and no American group had ever won.

That afternoon we competed, and I remember that we were really fired up. The Yale Glee Club had competed several years earlier and, I believe, had finished second. We were convinced that we had to at least equal the Yale club's performance.

And we did. We not only equaled them, we exceeded them and finished first, the first American singing group to do so. We were ecstatic. It was really a remarkable experience. That evening we sang some more American songs in the concert and performed really well. And then some of us went out to a Welsh pub and were entertained by some serious Welsh singing that was just awesome. I am a bass and I don't believe that I had ever heard the depth of bass voices that came out of that pub. But that does not take away from the fact that in our first performance in Europe, we had won the competition. And it was just a prelude to many enjoyable times in the two months to come in our tour visiting Scotland, London, Amsterdam, Bruges, Paris, Berlin, Copenhagen, Oslo, and Stockholm among others.

An equally enjoyable moment was having our group photograph taken in front of the Brandenburg Gate in Berlin. It was taken only shortly before the Berlin Wall was erected and the Brandenburg Gate was relegated to the control of the Russians in East Berlin.

The University of Michigan Men's Glee club was founded in 1857 and had a 150th reunion at Ann Arbor in the spring of 2010. A number of the members of the 1959 tour group to Wales showed up. It was a memorable occasion, since it was the 50th anniversary of that tour. Bob McGrath, who sang tenor in the club my junior year, and went on to fame as Bob in Sesame Street, was the emcee for an alumni concert on Saturday afternoon where about 450 alums showed up to sing. It was a very rewarding experience. I also was able to reconnect with Bob Ely, my colleague and singing partner of the "Admiral's Waiters" days aboard the USS Wisconsin.

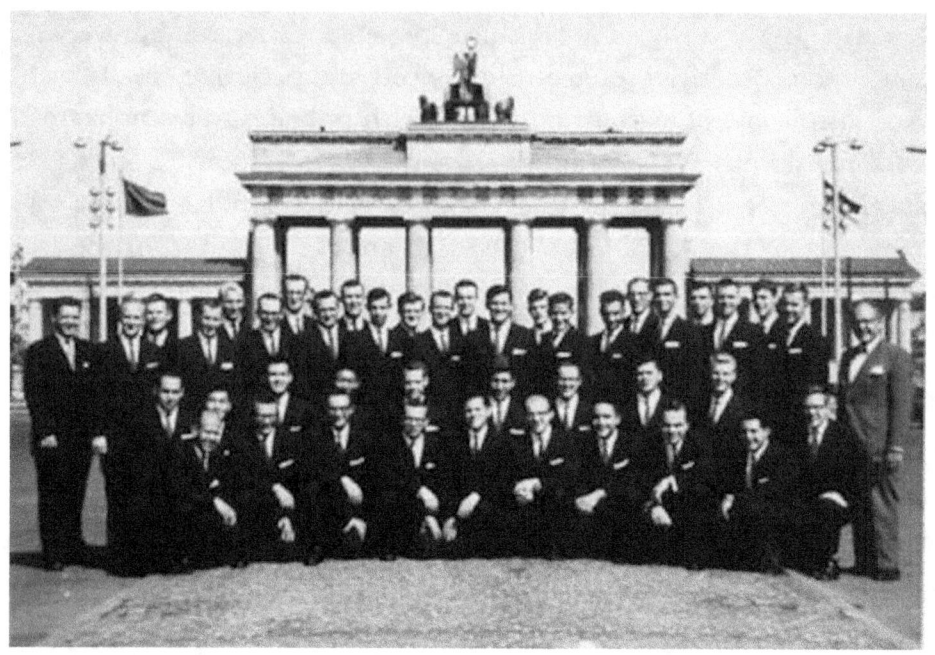

University of Michigan Men's Glee Club at Brandenburg Gate, 1959

CHAPTER 34
Jackson, Michigan, & the Ski Club

I returned from the University of Michigan Men's Glee Club tour to Europe, and joined IBM in the Dearborn, Michigan office on September 1, 1959. Shortly after, I was sent to Cleveland for my initial training class on punched cards, which took a couple of months. So about the middle of November, I showed up again at the Dearborn office. Most new recruits are assigned to work in punched card accounts. But since I had already studied computers at Michigan, I was not assigned a punched-card account, but an IBM tape 650 account at one of the Ford Motor Company locations in Birmingham, Michigan. It was a step up from the normal assignment. After about a month of this activity, I learned that I was moving again.

IBM was setting up a new program to assist large accounts in the installation of a new computer called the 7070. It was called Project Over-man. The IBM 7070 was to be the new flagship large computer system for commercial customers and there were to be a handful of these installations in the IBM Midwestern Region of the US, including Consumers Power Company in Jackson, Michigan; Michigan Bell Telephone in Detroit; and Dow Chemical in Midland, Michigan. Each account was to be "over-manned" by two IBM computer specialists for a period of eighteen months to assist in the installation of the computer systems. I interviewed for the program and learned that I was selected for the Consumers Power Company account.

So in January of 1960, I joined with the Jim Ricketts, other IBM representative being assigned to the account, and we went to Jackson, Michigan, the headquarters of the account, to meet the local IBM salesman and the customer executives there before heading off to Chicago for three months of intensive computer training on the IBM 7070. Little did I know at the time that my eighteen-month assignment would stretch into seven and a half years.

We had a very enjoyable class experience in Chicago. We stayed in the Allerton Hotel on Michigan Avenue where we could walk to the IBM class facilities on Pallister Avenue. We attended school during the day and then tried to hit a different restaurant each evening. And we normally followed that by a tour of Rush Street and other local haunts. Both Jim and I did well in the school so we were able to maximize our study of the local activities. Jim particularly liked the newly opened Playboy Club. We also liked the Embers Restaurant near Rush Street, as well as George Diamonds in downtown Chicago and some of the watering holes on West Elm Street.

Returning to Jackson in the spring, we found a rental property in a house at 5100 Browns Lake Road to share and proceeded to get to work. We were assigned tasks in the implementation plan as if we were employees and worked side by side with company staff. The consulting firm Arthur Andersen was also involved in the management of the project. The project was due to be completed in the summer of 1961.

Now we had to find some activities to fill our free time. Jim was a skier and checked out the local Jackson Ski Club. By the time we arrived in Jackson it was near the end of that year's ski season, but we found out that the club met once a week for social activities and went on one ski weekend a month during the season. Most of the trips were to ski locations in the upper part of the lower peninsula of Michigan, about a 4-5 hour car trip from Jackson. Jim was a good skier and hit many of the expert slopes. I had skied a couple of times before, but not seriously. I became a skier again as well; beginner level, and went along on many of the trips with my banjo in tow.

And the Consumers Power Project had moved into implementation stages so that was busy as well. So busy that, while Jim moved on to the Lansing office after his eighteen months was up, I was asked to stay on for another year, by both IBM and the customer. I was still a fairly new employee, but I was getting involved in some fairly heavy-duty stuff including becoming the IBM 1401 and 1410 expert in the office. And in that role I was being asked to visit other accounts in Michigan and Indiana as the "traveling expert." In January, 1963, I was also asked to take over as marketing representative at the Consumers Power Account and later that same year at Aeroquip, another large Jackson account. I was living the good life as a bachelor in Jackson, with a good job and a number of other activities.

Aeroquip had a Data Processing executive named Burleigh Cook, (no relation) who was very demanding of his IBM representatives and had a very creative and competent staff that required a lot of support.

He had a new IBM computer system on order and as part of the competitive bidding process had asked the vendors to write programs for their new computer systems. The IBM systems engineer that had written the program for Burleigh's bid had moved on to an overseas job, so I was asked by our branch manager to get the program working. I had to go to the Detroit datacenter to work on it, and after some extended effort to understand the program, which was written in an assembler language, I got it working. I don't think that Burleigh ever planned to use the completed program, he just wanted to know that the vendor could get it working.

We also later found out that the IBM configuration of the new computer system that he had ordered (a Disk Oriented IBM 1410 System) was not supported by the operating system that was being provided by IBM. Again I was asked to provide a solution, although this time I had to go to the Chicago Datacenter to get access to the information that I needed to get it resolved. It was a more complicated problem to solve and took me a couple of trips to Chicago, but I finally got it working. Aeroquip used my solution for a number of years. And Burleigh and IBM were both very grateful for my efforts.

It was on November 22, 1963 that I was in Burleigh's office, with an IBM specialist for the manufacturing industry from Chicago, when word came that President John F. Kennedy had been shot in Dallas, Texas. All work related activity stopped at that moment and we were all in a state of shock and disbelief. I don't think that many US adults would forget where they were on that day.

I learned years later that Burleigh had said that I was one of the best IBM representatives that he ever had. And I had enjoyed working with him as well. He was demanding but fair.

I had become a little better on skis and was going on many of the weekend ski trips. And it was on such a trip to the Boyne Mountain Lodge in January 1967 that I met the pretty girl in a red Bogner bonnet in the bar, whoops, I mean the lounge. She was from Royal Oak, Michigan and was there with some girl friends and we chatted for a bit one evening. I thought that she was one of the prettiest girls that I had ever met. But I was living in Jackson and she was living in the Detroit suburbs and I thought that my chances of seeing her again were somewhere between slim and none. And I didn't even get her name.

When I did eventually see her again, she admitted that since I had talked to her about "The Mikado", a Gilbert & Sullivan show that I was performing in at the time, she thought that I was Japanese.

I would have to say that between work and social activities, there were few dull moments in my life in Jackson, Michigan.

CHAPTER 35
The Clark Lake Players

I believe that my claim to fame in Jackson, Michigan was not just with IBM but with the Clark Lake Players as well. I had been in several plays in high school in Bowling Green, Ohio, and I found out that there was a very active summer playhouse on a lake about 15 miles south of Jackson. The playhouse itself was on the upper level of a two story building on the lake and the lower level was a restaurant/bar that was one of the local hangouts for the lake crowd.

The Clark Lake Players performed about five plays over the summer season, each running for two to three weeks (a week meaning the show was on Thurs/Fri/Sat). The opening play was normally one that had been successful on Broadway and ran for three weeks, while the closing play was usually a hit musical that also ran for three weeks. They had tryouts in May for the whole season and I went to the try out for the last production, the musical, South Pacific. The tryouts attracted performers from all over the area and some of the people had professional backgrounds.

I found out that the reigning leading man for many of the shows was Jerry Dixon, the local IBM typewriter salesman. He had an excellent baritone voice and looked the part of a leading man. I had been assigned to the Lansing, Michigan IBM office (home of Michigan State University, one of University of Michigan's top rivals) in conjunction with my project at Consumers Power Company, but found out that there was a local IBM sub-office in Jackson for the local IBM staff, and I had met Jerry there.

I did not expect to be competing for leading roles at that time, but over time I found Jerry stood in the way of some of the roles that I might want to play. Needless to say, I was accepted for a part in the chorus of South Pacific, and, while at audition, tried out for a part in Mister Roberts, the opening play. I got the part of Dolan, the sailor who brings a live goat onstage. We actually had a live goat and he (or she) and I became fast friends over the three weeks of the show. And Jerry, well, he was Mr. Roberts of course.

But it was a fun experience. Clark Lake was an active lake about seven miles long with a yacht club, an abundance of floating rafts, power boats for water skiing and a lot of summer cottages. The Clark Lake Players was an established area theatrical organization with professional direction, stage management, dual pianos for accompaniment, etcetera- a well-managed playhouse. The restaurant/bar on the floor below the playhouse attracted a lot of the area singles crowd, and there was another equally active bar on the opposite side of the lake. They were good stomping grounds for the area bachelors, me included.

Over the next six years, I performed in at least one play each summer, sometimes two, and really enjoyed the experience. After that first summer experience with Mr. Roberts & South Pacific, I performed in Pajama Game, Annie Get Your Gun, Kiss Me Kate (had the part of Gremio), and Brigadoon (with another theater group), among others. Jerry Dixon was the male lead in many of them. I wasn't getting any lead roles, but I was developing theatrical skills.

And then something happened. Jerry got promoted to the IBM office in San Francisco; and he took the job, so he was not going to be around for the 1965 season. That was my chance. The opening play of that season was the "Fantasticks," which at the time was a long running off-Broadway play in NYC. I tried out for and got the part of El Gallo, the Narrator. A juicy role.

I had to work hard on it, but I did a good enough job through the nine performances at Clark Lake that I was offered the same role in the Jackson Winter Theater 18 months later. I finally had grabbed a lead role and had done it well, and that led to more roles in more theatre groups.

There was a Gilbert & Sullivan Society in the local Methodist church where the choir director also directed the plays. I parlayed my experience at Clark Lake into several roles there. I did the Pirate King in the "Pirates of Penzance," Pooh Bah in "The Mikado," and had major roles in "The Gondaliers" and "Iolanthe." I also had a nice role in "A Funny Thing Happened on the Way to the Forum" at Clark Lake. So I was now a respected actor in the local theatre groups and could try out for the roles that I wanted.

Between work, the ski club and the theater I was quite busy, and still had time for the Junior Chamber of Commerce (Jaycees), where I served a year as a director. I also had time to serve as a groomsman in my younger brother Dan's wedding in the summer of 1966. But the varied theater groups in Jackson, Michigan gave me an excellent opportunity to develop my theatrical talents.

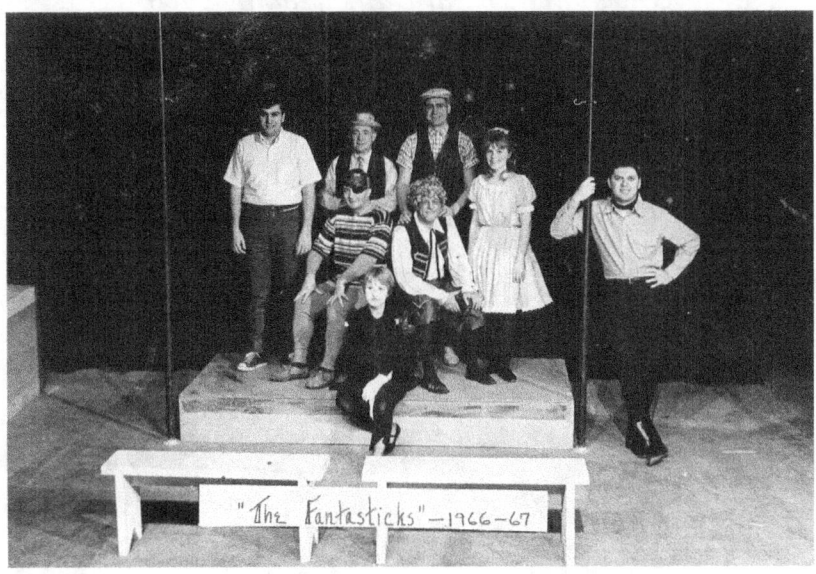

"The Fantasticks"

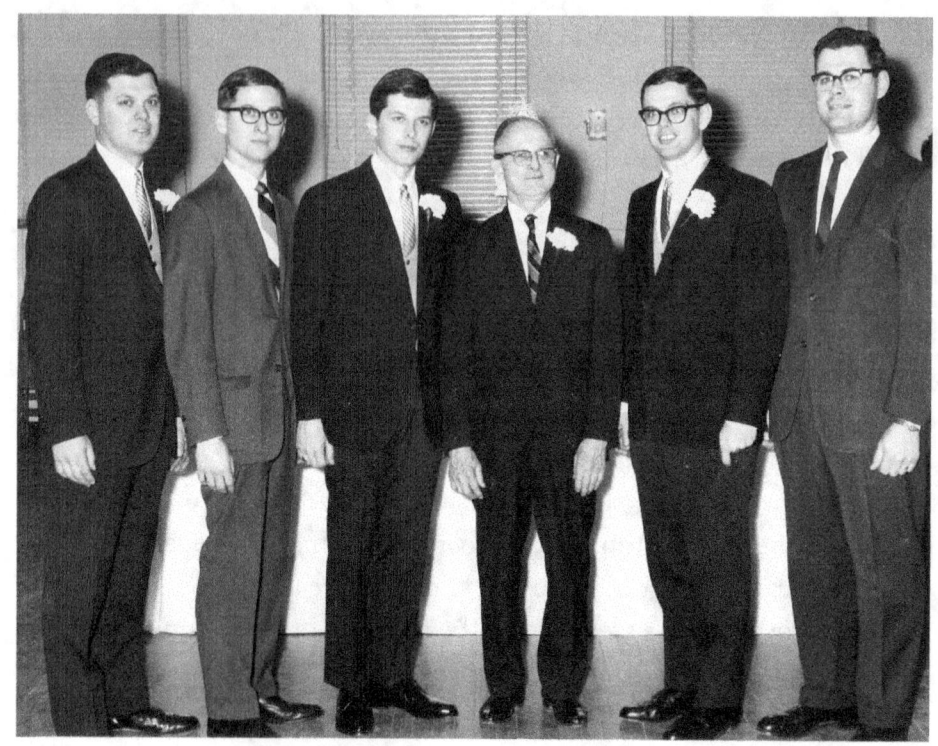

Gilbert and sons at Dan's wedding-1966

CHAPTER 36
"Grab the Ring, Boy"

Our office was part of the IBM Detroit District and our district manager was a former Marine by the name of "Boomer" Page. I never knew his real first name. To us troops he was just "Boomer" and if you had ever heard him talk you would know how he got that name. He could have been a drill sergeant; and maybe he once was.

Well, we were having a sub-office meeting in Jackson one day in the spring of 1967 and "Boomer" was in attendance, which should have given me a clue that something was going on, but it didn't. Then at the end of the meeting, I was asked if I would mind driving Boomer up to Lansing so he could attend another meeting there. It was not something that I could refuse, so a bit later, Boomer and I were in my car driving the 45 minutes or so up to Lansing. IBM had a fairly hierarchal organization those days and salesmen rarely talked directly to district managers, but went through the chain of command via the branch manager. This day turned out to be an exception to that rule.

A few miles along the highway "Boomer" turned to me and said in his normal voice which was, to put it mildly, loud and booming. "Well, Wayne, I guess you know why I want to talk to you." I about smashed up the car. Not only had I not talked to him about anything before, but I did I not have a clue about why he would want to talk to me now.

He went on to explain that they were having some competitive problems with the Burroughs Corporation at the Michigan Bell Telephone account, which was the largest IBM account in the Detroit Commercial Office. It seemed that Burroughs was a Detroit-based company, and one of the senior executives at Michigan Bell was on the board of Burroughs and vice-versa. Burroughs had just announced a new computer system that was capable of taking over the entire Michigan Bell IBM account.

He wanted me to move to the Detroit Commercial office and take over as lead salesman on the team. The team would include about a dozen marketing representatives and systems engineers. I had just tried out for one of the leads in the musical Camelot at Clark Lake, which was a role that I had been eager to get. And I didn't know how to respond to Boomer. I happened to know several members of the Michigan Bell team, including one who had been a fraternity brother at Michigan, and I wanted to talk to them before I had to make a decision.

Boomer told me to "Grab the ring, boy. Grab the ring" referring to the rings on a merry-go-round. I was at a loss for words. He also said that while it would be considered a lateral move, there would be a salary increase that came with it. It would be for eighteen months (just like my eighteen month move to Jackson was, ha ha) and would be considered the equivalent of staff experience. In IBM at the time, staff experience was normally a requirement to moving from a sales job to marketing manager, which is the first job in the management chain. I told Boomer that I appreciated the opportunity and that I would like to get back to him.

After driving Boomer to the office where he was going to make some sales calls, I went to talk to my Branch Manager, and asked him what he knew about the situation. He said from what he knew, it was a very competitive account and Boomer was being pressured to find some new blood, including a new lead salesman. My manager didn't know much else, but he was prepared to let me go. Knowing how IBM works, I don't think he had much choice.

Well, about a week later I got a call from Tom Nebel, the Branch Manager of the IBM Detroit Commercial branch office asking "Where are you?" I set up an appointment to meet with him in Detroit. He first words were "Where have you been? You are already on my payroll." And he went on to explain the situation at the account. I asked him if it was OK for me to go to see Boomer and he agreed. So I drove out to the District Office, about 5 miles north of the branch office. The Assistant District Manager, who was well versed on the situation, met me and told me that Boomer was tied up in a meeting at that time, but that Boomer really wanted me to take the job. I said "Do I have a choice?." And he said "Not really."

So a few weeks later, in the summer of 1967, I was on my way to Detroit with much of my stuff in the back seat and trunk of my car on the way to a motel down the street from the IBM Detroit Commercial office. I had been selected to play one of the leads in Camelot and had to tell the director that I was not going to be able to do it. The office had appointed a replacement for me at my accounts and I had made the necessary hand-over calls. When we made the turn-over call on the Chairman of Consumers Power Company, he said "IBM can replace you as our salesman, but what are the Clark Lake Players going to do?" which I took as a sincere compliment to both my IBM and my acting abilities.

And I thought that maybe, just maybe, I might run into the girl that I had met at Boyne Mountain earlier in the year.

So there I was. Driving along on a Sunday afternoon on I-94, one of Detroit's freeways, whistling a tune, when I noticed something unusual. There were no cars on the road. I was the only one. Then I saw some national guard trucks loaded with troops, and thought "this is not good news." I did not have the radio on but immediately turned it on.

I was driving into Detroit on one of the days of the 1967 riots. All cars off of the road, and the motel where I was to stay at was in the middle of the riot district. So I decided on an alternate plan, high-tailed it off of the main road and hunkered down at a different motel until the next day.

The next morning, standing on the roof of the Michigan Bell Telephone building with some of my new IBM teammates as well as some Michigan Bell employees, we looked toward downtown Detroit and watched the smoke rise. The IBM Detroit Commercial Branch Office was located right in the middle of the riot area.

———————————

Then it happened. It was only a few weeks later when I was at a Young Republican social event at the Roostertail Restaurant, which was located along the Detroit River. I was walking upstairs for some reason, and there she was, the girl that I had met at Boyne Mountain, walking downstairs with a girlfriend. Just like in the movies. We passed on the stairs and I nodded. She moved on.

I asked one of my IBM friends, Roger Sargeant, if he knew who she was, and he told me that she was a good friend of a girl living in the same apartment building that he lived in and that he could get me her phone number. Roger said that her name was Patricia Poser and she was a school teacher. And my gut told me that I wanted to marry her.

I had just turned 34 years old that July, I was entering into a new phase at IBM and it was probably about time that I settled down.

Consumers Power NEWS

Photo Report to Stockholders: April, 1967 for the 19th Consecutive Series of Regional Stockholder Meetings

News of Expansion and Progress in Electronics, Nuclear Power and Electric and Gas System Operations—All Designed to Meet Growing Demands for Energy in Michigan.

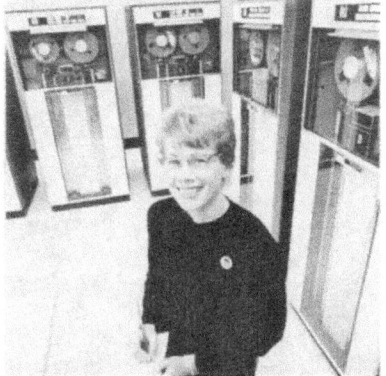

Six New Computer Systems Being Added Over Two-Year Period

Consumers Power Company's electronic computer facilities are being substantially expanded to increase operating efficiencies, improve customer service and sharpen operating controls and engineering planning. Four major new computer systems were added in 1966. Two more are scheduled for 1967, the first of which already has been received. Four of these six new systems are additions to the electronic data processing program. Two are process control computers, one assigned to electric operations and the other to gas system operations. At left, a competent (and pretty) secretary poses before electronic tape processors, suggesting pictorially that the Company combines capable people and modern facilities to provide high-quality energy services. Below, a new electronic unit is inspected during installation.

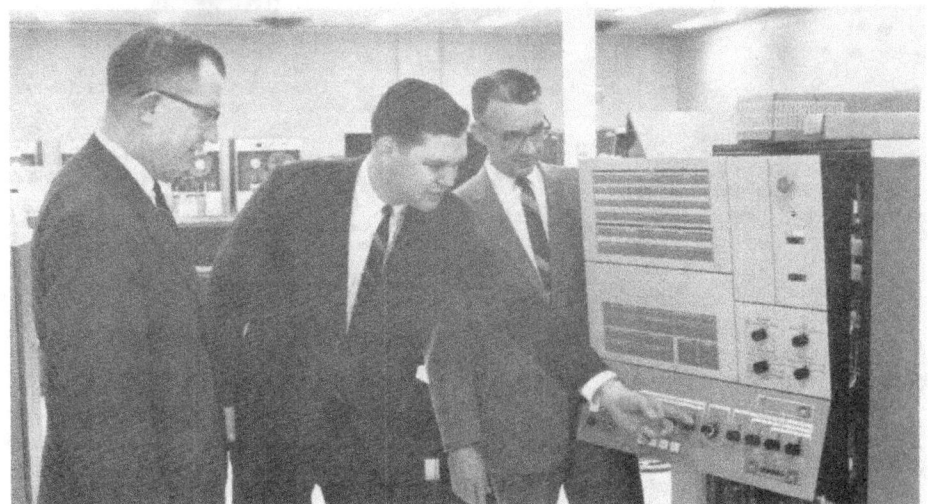

Consumers Power Company-1967

CHAPTER 37
Dating in Detroit

I called Pat Poser, the girl that I had seen at the Roostertail Restaurant, up for a date, and she was busy. I asked for a date further out. She was still busy. So I asked if she was interested in getting together at all. She admitted that for the next month she was traveling the state of Michigan as Miss Michigan Young Republican supporting George Romney in his bid for the presidency. So I accepted that as a reasonable alternative to going out with me, and we did set a date to get together after her stint with Romney.

We had a good time on that first date and set another date. And another. But IBM started to intervene. As part of my work with Michigan Bell Telephone, we had an installation of an IBM 360 Model 65 computer system going on in their datacenter in Port Huron, Michigan, and it was not going well. This was a computer system announced in April 1964 that was intended as the replacement for the 7070. It was an early installation, not only for Michigan Bell but for the entire Bell System, and if it did not go smoothly it did not bode well for IBM installations all across the US. So it was a very visible installation, and we had to make it work.

I won't go into the problems that we had, but what we did to help solve it was set up an old-fashioned Navy watch bill. The installation was scheduled to run programs round the clock. We set up three eight- hour shifts with a responsible IBMer on each shift, and I was the overall lead rep. We scheduled daily reviews at the start of the 8 AM shift. We also had access to competent Michigan Bell staff. They wanted to solve the problems as much as we did.

This basically meant that I moved to a hotel in Port Huron for about a month and made myself available 24 hours a day while we resolved the main issues of the problem. This also meant that I was not able to see Pat as much as I would have liked and had to find time to sneak down from Port Huron when possible. But we finally did get the installation running smoothly. I was able to establish excellent working relationships with many of the Michigan Bell staff as a result. And we received plaudits from the national IBM industry representatives as well.

I took Pat down to Bowling Green, Ohio to see my parents at their new home on Ranch Court and that Thanksgiving we went to my brother Dean's house in Kalamazoo, where he was teaching chemistry at Western Michigan University. My brothers, Al and Jim, were both married and living in apartments in the Bronx area of New York City at the time, and they invited us to visit them. So over Christmas 1967, we decided to go to New York City. The IBM office arranged to order the tickets for me. To cover up the personal nature of the trip, Pat's name on her ticket was TC Wayne. My parents decided to join us and we elected to see the Nutcracker at Lincoln Center as one of our events.

It was that evening, as Pat and I walked back to Jim's apartment after the performance, that I asked her to marry me and gave her a ring. She accepted. It was a wonderful end to the evening and to our New York City trip.

After that things moved along pretty quickly. We planned for a June 1968 wedding at the Shrine of the Little Flower, the Catholic Church that she and her parents attended. In the middle of our plans, IBM intervened again, but this time in a more positive way.

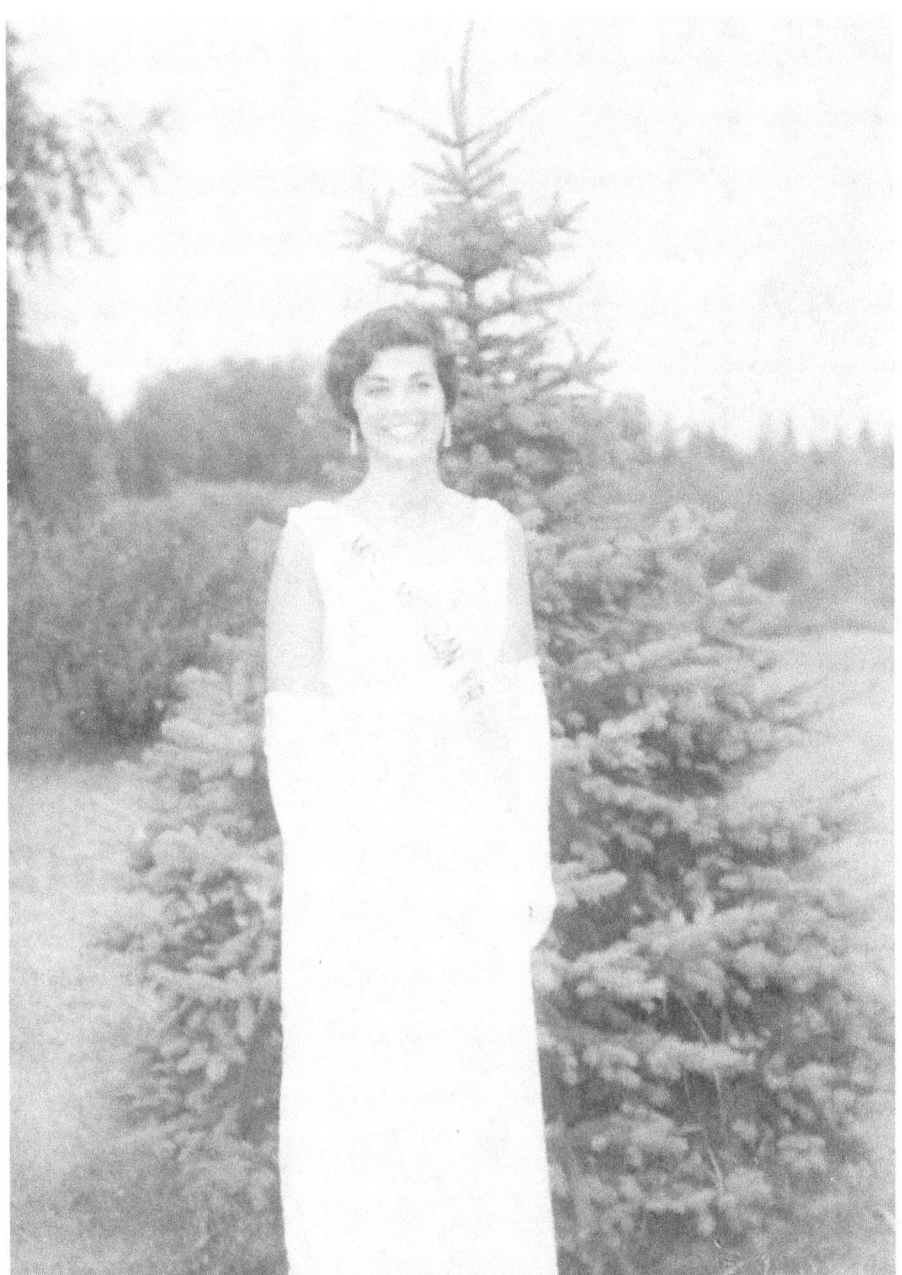

Pat Poser, Miss Michigan Young Republican-1967

CHAPTER 38
"Captain IBM"

Shortly after the first of the year in 1968, I was asked to try out for the IBM Midwestern Region 100% Club Players, a group of five IBMers from around the Region, who were going to perform for the 100% Club being held at the Palmer House Hotel in Chicago in April. Two singers from Detroit (myself, and John Sirich, from the GM office), one from Minneapolis, and two from Chicago started rehearsal in Chicago for the club. It was a three-day recognition event for the top performers in the Region for the previous year. Due to my move to Detroit in the middle of the previous year, I had not qualified for that year's club. We were to have an opening number on each day, a coffee break number each day, and on the last day a mini-review with a collection of numbers.

We had two full weeks of solid rehearsal in Chicago prior to the event, which was coordinated by two ex-Broadway types and had original music and a full orchestra. I originally had one solo number as a Gilbert and Sullivan type song announcing the arrival the District Manager. But there was another solo number as Captain IBM, and the person originally selected to sing it turned down the role. I was asked to step in. It was a real campy song with a cape. I had to enter the stage from behind a ribbon screen with a microphone connected to a wireless transmitter that was stuck in the back of my waist, an early use of technology that is commonplace today.

It worked ok during rehearsal, but, during the show, I got a little excited entering the stage from behind the ribbon screen, stretched my arms out when entering and pulled the microphone cord out of the wireless transmitter. I was onstage with no mike. But as they say, the show must go on, and I sang as loud as I could to make up for it in front of a full audience of about 300 people.

All of the performers except me were married, and their wives were invited to come to the show at IBM's expense. At the last minute it was decided that Pat should come as well, and she did, and was able to experience an IBM 100% Club first hand. They needed to give her a name badge and the one that they gave her said that it was her eighth club. IBM booked us in separate rooms, of course.

At the opening show, we were all garbed up with matching outfits and stage makeup. Our outfits included grey single-breasted suits, blue blazers and grey flannel slacks, which IBM paid for and gave us, as well as the white shirts and neckties. So IBM helped me recoup from some of my earlier mistakes with buying clothes. These were nice looking outfits that I had for some time.

After the first show, the vibes from the audience were that we were all professionals hired by IBM just for the event. So to alter the look, we dropped the stage makeup for the rest of the performances and an announcement was made about who we actually were. The rest of the performances went on without a hitch.

After the last performance, it was suggested that we should go back to Chicago and record an album of the show. And we did just that a couple of weeks later at a professional Chicago sound stage replete with an orchestra. It was an interesting experience, just like you see in the movies. The five of us in a soundproof room, watching the conductor through a window, and listening to the orchestra, which we could see was playing, but could hear only through our headphones.

The vinyl records were sent to all of the attendees. And I recently learned that a handful of the songs have been loaded into the Internet, and are available for your listening pleasure at www.park.org/cdrom/ pavilions/IBM/percentclub.

It was a wonderful experience for both Pat and me and I was able to make full use of my musical skills.

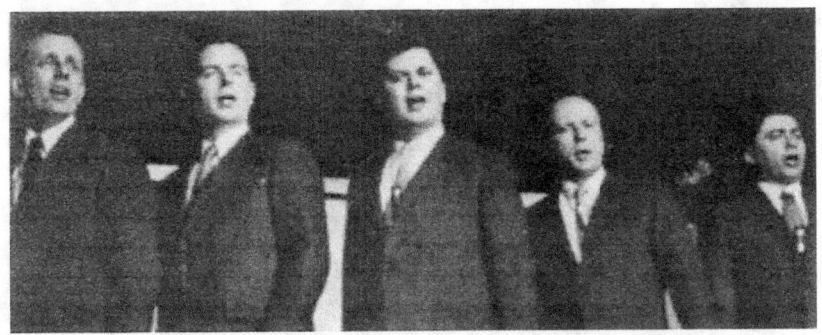

IBM Hundred Percent Club Quintet-1968

CHAPTER 39
Life in Somerset Park

We got married on June 22, 1968. My brother, Dan, was my best man and Pat's brothers, Bob and Buzz, my brother, Dean, and an IBM friend, Larry Lauterbach, were my groomsmen. We honeymooned in Ocho Rios and Montego Bay, Jamaica and had a wonderful time.

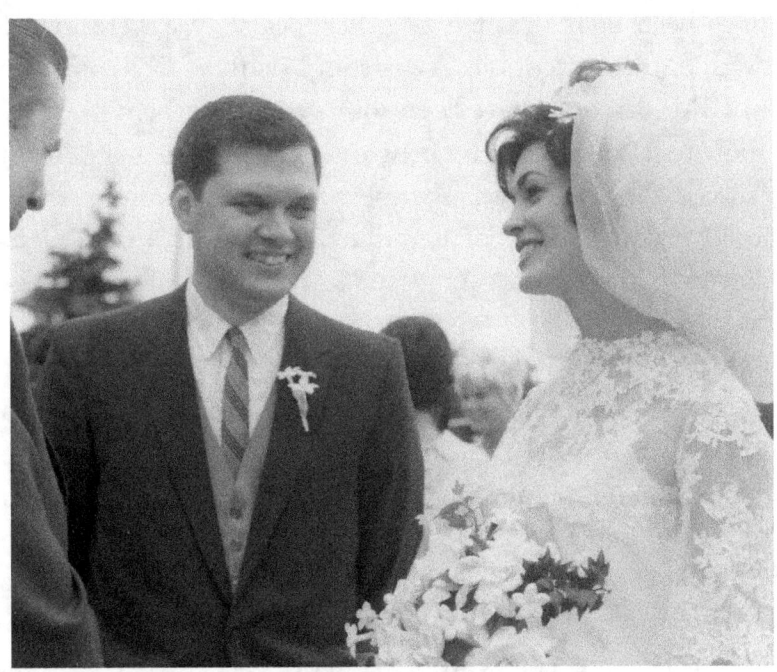

At Our Wedding-June 1968

When we arrived back at our new digs at an apartment in Somerset Park, in Troy, Michigan, (where I had previously been living with an IBM roommate) we got a new surprise. We had had a pretty bumpy flight back from Miami and Pat was not feeling so well.

When we opened the door to the bathroom, it was completely filled with paper. Filled. To the ceiling with rolled up newspapers. It took us a while to clean it out to discover that the water was turned off as well. We did get that resolved in short order, but throughout the following week, many little things cropped up. The stereo had been rewired. Liquor bottles switched around. All sorts of little gremlin-like things.

We tried to think about who would have done it and how they would have gotten into the apartment. A check of the newspapers used to fill the bathroom indicated that they were from the Detroit area so it was unlikely to have been any of my relatives, although it could have been Pat's brothers or other locals. We were in a dinner group with four other couples, two from Michigan Bell, and two others from IBM. It could have been some, or all, of them.

It took us about three months of investigative work before we finally solved the case. It was the members of the dinner group, who had convinced our next-door neighbor to let them in to leave some "gifts" for us. And it took about the same length of time to get the apartment back in order.

We started enjoying life in Detroit. Pat was busy with her job teaching speech and English at the local Troy High School, and we got into the Birmingham Village Players, a local theater group that was performing "Guys and Dolls." Pat landed a role as one of the "Hatbox Girls" and I was "Rusty Charlie," one of the gamblers and one of the trio that sings the opening number, "Fugue for Tinhorns." It was a lot of fun and we met a lot of new people from the area in the process. The Detroit Tigers won the World Series that year and the city seemed to be on a roll.

But at the end of the year, IBM reorganized. I had been told by "Boomer" that my eighteen months of work at Michigan Bell Telephone would be the equivalent of my staff experience prior to management. But as part of the reorganization, "Boomer" Page was no longer my district manager. The new district manager, Ed Frick, had offices located on Wacker Drive in downtown Chicago, and he did not believe in promoting managers directly from the field. He said that while he had heard about the excellent work that I had done at Michigan Bell Telephone, I would first have to go on his staff in Chicago before being considered for a management slot. I accepted a position as a district representative for the Utility and Communications Industries working remotely out of the Detroit office.

After a couple of months of traveling around the territory, which went from Cleveland to Minneapolis to Kansas City, I was asked if I wanted to sing again in the 100% club being held that year in Miami. And I actually attended a rehearsal in Princeton, NJ, of all places, of the group that was going to be performing.

But I was pre-empted by a call by Ed Frick to a meeting in Chicago regarding the Commonwealth Edison account. It was the public utility servicing the Chicago area and one of the largest accounts in Chicago. They were having performance problems with one of their systems, an IBM 360 Model 65, and Ed asked me to take over as the project manager to resolve the problem. Michigan Bell Telephone revisited.

So I started flying to Chicago on the first Monday morning flight from the local Detroit downtown airport to Meggs Field in downtown Chicago and returned on the late afternoon flight on Friday. In between, I was at Commonwealth Edison every morning for an IBM/customer meeting and was setting up various support teams during the day. Having been married just about eight months, it was kind of a strain, but I did not have much of a choice. And Pat & I managed through it.

I did offer up a replacement for the 100% Club show: my brother, Dan, who was working for IBM in Cincinnati. He was contacted, took the role and enjoyed it very much.

The marketing manager of the Commonwealth Edison account when I started working there was named Larry Chapman, and about half way through my project, he was promoted to Branch Manager of the Pittsburgh Gateway office. It was probably a good idea to have him move on from the Commonwealth Edison account, since he would then not need to be involved in any solutions that we proposed.

We successfully finished the Commonwealth project in about a month and a half, during which I was able to re-orient myself to Chicago. I had actually spent a weekend with Larry Lauterbach, who had been in my wedding party, and was now working for IBM in Chicago, looking at possible areas in which to live in Chicago.

And at the end of my Chicago project, my manager there offered me up a free ticket to Miami, where the 100% Club had been held, as a compromise for the work that I had done and the fact that I had not been able to sing at the club in Miami. Pat and I parlayed that into two tickets to Nassau in the Bahamas and had a fun week there. One highlight was seeing Aristotle Onassis' boat coming in to dock with Onassis and a gaggle of Kennedys on board, including Jacqueline.

Shortly after we returned from that trip, one of the marketing managers in Larry Chapman's new office in Pittsburgh left IBM for personal reasons and Larry needed to hire a new marketing manager for the utility and insurance accounts. The next week I found myself in a hotel in Gateway Center, Pittsburgh, interviewing for the job. I probably had an inside track since I already had met Larry and had in effect already worked for him on the Commonwealth Edison project, so he knew what I could do. In any case, I got the job, and in July 1969, Pat and I found ourselves house-hunting and then moving to Pittsburgh, Pennsylvania. We moved into our first home at 1548 King Charles Drive in the North Hills of Pittsburgh the week that the astronauts walked on the moon. And there was additional excitement in our lives: Pat was expecting our first child.

CHAPTER 40
Pittsburgh, Pennsylvania

Pittsburgh was a great place to live and raise a family. No, seriously. We found the people very friendly, my work went well, and we had two children born at the local hospital, first our son Scott, and then, three years later, our daughter, Kelly. I didn't do a lot of overnight travelling with my job and the area IBM district office was just a couple of hours away in Cleveland, so we were able to get involved in local activities. We settled in, joined a swim club and started to enjoy life and our children.

There was a systems engineer in the IBM office where I worked, named Frank Hrach, who was a member of a men's barbershop-type singing chorus of about 50 voices called the Allegheny Good Tyme Singers. He asked me if I would like go to some of the rehearsals with him. I went, auditioned, was accepted and joined the group. We rehearsed once a week and also performed about once a week around Western Pennsylvania. We also had a couple of benefit concerts for the Big Brothers in Heinz Hall in downtown Pittsburgh, where we did the opening numbers and then had a name group perform the primary concert. We raised a lot of money for the charity and it was great fun to sing in Heinz Hall that had just been renovated.

I next joined a theater group called the North Star Players and ended up with nice roles in "The King and I," and "The Boy Friend." And Pat joined the group as well and got a role in "Oliver," so we were both busy with theater activities.

Frank Hrach then asked me if I would be interested in forming a quartet with him and two other members of the AGTS. I agreed and we started rehearsing for the annual barbershop quartet competition. We called ourselves "The Contemporaries" and made the cut of ten quartets in the first primary in Pittsburgh. But I was getting too busy with chorus rehearsals in addition to the quartet rehearsals and the theater activities.. And then we learned that Pat was pregnant again, so I told Frank that I could not continue through to the next competition in Cleveland. He understood and we terminated the quartet

After a couple of years with smaller IBM utility and insurance accounts, I was rewarded with the responsibility for the Mellon Bank account, which was the largest account in the office. It had a very knowledgeable and vocal IT executive named George DiNardo, who required a deft touch in managing. It was interesting that in my IBM career, I had been involved with the largest accounts in four different branch offices in the Midwest Region and had survived all of them: Consumers Power Company in Jackson, Michigan; Michigan Bell Telephone Company in Detroit; Commonwealth Edison in Chicago, and Mellon Bank in Pittsburgh. And in each account I had been involved with an IBM System 360 Model 65.

Pat and I joined a group that performed in a dinner theater at the local Methodist Church. It was there that we had one of our most enjoyable theater experiences, playing the lead roles of Giles and Molly Ralston in Agatha Christie's memorable play, "The Mousetrap." Our director was named Harriet Woodcock, and she was a professional. It may have been a church play, but it was a first class show with an excellent cast. We had early rehearsals in our basement since our daughter, Kelly, was a baby at the time. And we were in the middle of the performances at the time of my next promotion with IBM.

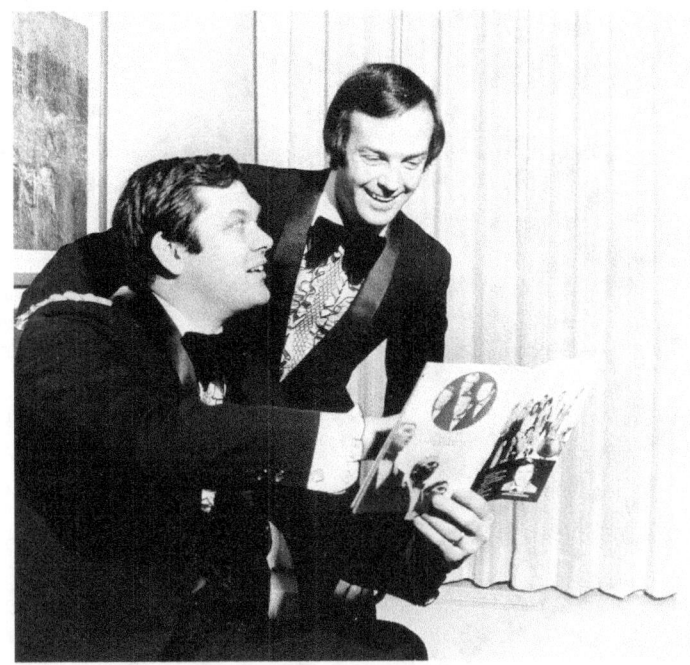

With Frank Hrach- Allegheny Good Tyme Singers-1971

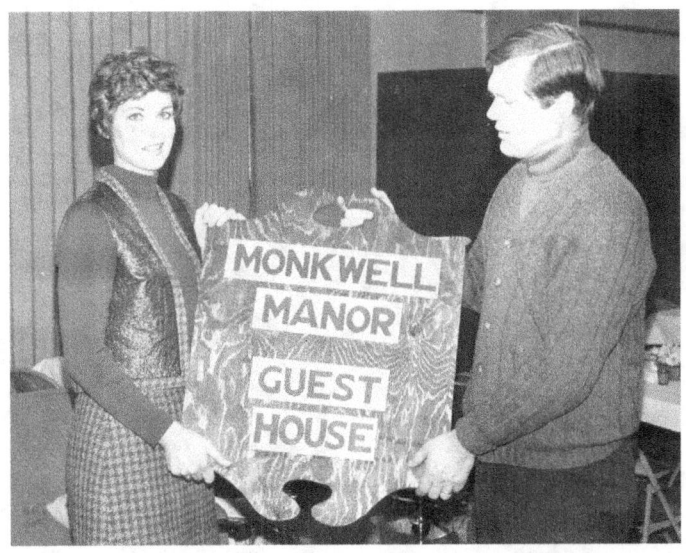

With Pat in "The Mousetrap"-1973

CHAPTER 41
Princeton, New Jersey

After four and a half years at the IBM Pittsburgh Gateway office, I was ready to move on. I had talked to my manager about options for new positions and he mentioned two possibilities: the telecommunications industry headquartered outside of Raleigh, North Carolina, and the banking industry located just outside of Princeton, New Jersey.

So I was not surprised when in the fall of 1973 I was asked to have a meeting with the director of banking industry marketing. He was going to be at a meeting in Boston, and I was to fly there to meet him at his hotel. We had a short meeting there, and he offered me a job in Princeton. The only problem was that he wanted me to start right away and I was in the middle of performances of the Mousetrap. I worked out a plan that I thought would be acceptable to enable me to make all of the performances and accepted the job. The problem with my plan was that I had not counted on the snow storm that I related on pages 14 and 15 of my first book, *On the Far Side of the Curve*. My car was parked at the Pittsburgh airport and it was completely covered with snow. But things worked out ok. And the show went on- on time.

It turned out the move had a couple of interesting twists to it. I was going to replace Dix Gedney as a Finance Industry Manager. And the job that I was leaving at Mellon Bank was being enhanced to an Account Executive position and Dix was going to replace me in that role. So we were in effect swapping jobs, and it was considered a promotion for us both.

My wife, Pat, had taken a liking to Dix's house at 43 Beech Hill Circle in Princeton, which was not yet on the market. So just prior to leaving Princeton to go home for Thanksgiving, Dix and I got together in his living room and worked out an agreement for our purchase of his house, which we did. We moved to Princeton in January 1974, and we have owned the home ever since.

By the time that I moved to Princeton, the Industry Director who had hired me had moved on and was replaced by John Bishop from New York City. Off and on over the next fifteen years, I would work for John on three continents.

CHAPTER 42
J. Paddington Poole

The IBM Finance Industry Marketing management job was a very busy one. At the time there were four managers reporting to John Bishop, the industry director. We had responsibility for IBM's domestic banking business spread from coast to coast: The strategy, the sales plan, marketing of the banking products, the education of the sales and systems engineering force, the coordination with the manufacturing facilities, the customer programs, the business shows, the advertising campaigns, the management of the Industry Specialist program. You name it. We worked on it. We spent a lot of time in meetings both in Princeton and around the country with both the local IBMers and the customer executives, so there was a lot of travel with the job. There were also a number of trouble-shooting calls. But I enjoyed it and believe that I did it well. Then John Bishop came to me with a special assignment.

It was the spring of 1975 and we had just announced a number of enhancements to our 3600 banking terminal product line. The American Banking Association had its annual meeting scheduled for Oahu, Hawaii that summer with thousands of expected attendees. John wanted to do something big to hype the product line and he wanted me to put it together. John was concerned about the time we had to get it done and encouraged me to develop a comprehensive work plan for his periodic review.

We got in contact with a marketing company in New York City and started work. By the time we were ready to leave for Hawaii we had prepared a half hour large screen presentation using five slide projectors and a live presenter. It could handle an audience of several hundred. It was the most comprehensive presentation that we had ever attempted. The work-plan had worked- so far.

The concept dealt with a gentleman called J. Paddington Poole who lived in a town that had a number of businesses that were interconnected in thought but not actually and about how the new IBM systems could enable all of the businesses to communicate with each other. An excellent idea but, as it turned out, we were ahead of our time. We were not able to fund the entire cost of the show out of our own business show budget and had gotten financial support from a number of other IBM headquarters organizations.

As you might imagine, we had a team of people involved in putting on the show; the staff from the marketing company, the presenters, our IBM staff, the IBM business show staff, etcetera. And we arrived in Hawaii, went through our dress rehearsals and got ready to go. We had a theater set up to handle the crowds.

And then something funny happened. Well not really. It was not really funny. It was something that we probably should have thought about but got lost in our enthusiasm to create the show. Nobody showed up. Well not "nobody," but not the crowds that we expected.

We checked with the other companies that had scheduled events at the meetings; demonstrations, presentations, and other activities and found that the same thing was happening to other computer companies as well. Except most of the other companies had not gone to the extent and expense that we had.

But the bankers were not going to the meetings and seminars, they were going to the beach. They were using the ABA event as a paid vacation and most of them had brought their wives and were enjoying the beaches and restaurants of Hawaii.

And we were left with an expensive show with only a little response to show for it.

I was mortified and embarrassed. John met with me to discuss what we could do. Well, we came up with a plan to revise the presentation materials to make them work in a smaller environment so that we could use them in our executive briefings and other presentations. It was not what we had intended but it worked. And I had to come up with a presentation to take to the other organizations that had helped fund us to show them how they could get some value out of what we had done. I also had to give a private showing of the revised presentation to our industry vice president.

All of that worked and we were able to get through the aftermath unscathed. But John used that event to highlight one of his numerous "Bishopisms." "The acceptance of an idea is more important than the quality." Touché.

And actually, over time, the concept that we used in the "J. Paddington Poole" presentation came to be an important part of the IBM offerings in the concept known as EFTS- Electronic Funds Transfer Systems. We were just a few years ahead of ourselves. And I kept my job.

CHAPTER 43
"1776"

At the end of 1975, after surviving J. Paddington Poole, I thought that I had a pretty good handle on my job and could take the time to be in a play. I tried out for a play to be performed at the local McCarter Theater in Princeton, along with one of my neighbors, Herb Horowitz. It was "1776" to be performed in January 1976. I got a part as a southern senator from North Carolina, Joseph Hewes, who at the time of the American Revolution had owned a home in Princeton, actually not far from my own home. It was a singing part with only a few lines involved. Herb got the part of a Senator Bartlett from Massachusetts.

In the summer of 1975, after returning from the ABA National in Hawaii, I had been asked to be in an IBM "task force," a small group of people who got together to create solutions for specific problems that were outside of the normal organization. The one that I worked on was looking at solutions to the pricing and marketing of IBM industry specific products in the banking and retail store system organizations to find ways to be more price-competitive.

We had spent a couple of months looking at the problems and had developed a comprehensive flip chart presentation with issues, recommendations and organization plans. We had left the presentation at one of the IBM offices in White Plains. We actually got approval for pilot implementations in Baltimore and San Francisco, but approval for a full rollout was deferred.

Then, in January 1976, I was asked to rejoin the task force and plan for a national rollout. Unfortunately, it was at a time that we were having daily rehearsals for the play, which was due to start performances the end of January. To make matters worse, since the majority of the task force members were located in White Plains, New York, that was where we were to meet.

The first order of business was to find the old charts, where we had summarized the objectives, issues, recommendations, US organization, implementation plan, etcetera. The White Plains administrators unsuccessfully looked for them for a couple of days. If we did not find the charts, we would have had to re-do a lot of our previous work.

Then one day I was in the IBM office in White Plains where the charts were last seen and had the inspiration that maybe they had fallen behind one of the filing cabinets. So we looked behind all of the filing cabinets and, lo and behold, there they were, lying in a pile behind one of the cabinets just waiting to be found. We could now start work again from where we had left off. It created a good feeling for the task force members.

For most of January, I was getting up early in the morning, driving to the IBM office in White Plains, spending the day in task force mode, driving two hours back to Princeton, stopping by the house to catch a bite and then heading for rehearsals, which lasted until 11 or so. And I was keeping my normal job under control at the same time. The director of the play was an experienced Broadway type. It was probably the most professionally run play that I had ever experienced. Several of the cast members were card-carrying professionals or had been involved with the "soaps" in NYC.

The rehearsals were all conducted in a professional manner. If you missed a rehearsal without a reason, you were out. And if you were late too many times, you were out. Once I was late and got a really good chewing out, so I made sure that did not happen again. But as my wife, Pat, will tell you, for that month I ran on fumes. I don't know how I appeared everywhere I was supposed to be on time, but I did. The play was a success. And the task force recommendations were accepted; a separate sales force for the financial and retail store system products was established along with a new pricing methodology and a unique quota system. Success all the way around. Using my talents in planning as well as acting had come into play.

CHAPTER 44
The Cottage at Island Lake

Mickey and Charlie Poser, Pat's parents, owned a home in Royal Oak, Michigan, as well as several rental properties in the area. They also owned a cottage on Island Lake, located about 45 minutes outside of Royal Oak close to Brighton, Michigan. The cottage was larger than your typical lake cottage with living room, dining room, kitchen, and three bedrooms. But the thing that made it special for our children, Scott and Kelly, was the front screened in porch that had four cots for sleeping. They slept there most of the time that we visited, which was often. I would say that over the years from the time the kids were born until we went to Hong Kong in 1986, they were at the cottage sometime during every year.

It was called Island Lake because there was an island in the middle of the lake that you could get to by boat, or even swimming, if you took your time. There was also a state park on the lake with typical park operations.

At another nearby park on Kent Lake, the Posers had a food stand that they operated in the summer that sold pop, hamburgers, hot dogs, etcetera, that was open on the weekends. They also had a canoe rental where you could schedule a pick-up at several selected spots along a river. Mr. Poser and his two boys, Buzz and Bob, were kept busy on the weekends with canoe drop offs and pickups. So Island and Kent Lake were busy places, particularly on the weekends.

The cottage had a historical background since it had been the living quarters for the bands that used to play in the '30s and '40s in the dance hall pavilion on the point next to the cottage. The dance hall was a big draw in the area with a lot of the big bands of the era coming to play. The pavilion had burned down years ago and was never replaced, but the cottage endured.

The cottage was right on the lake and down a short ways from a swimming hole and dock. Swimming was always a large part of going to the lake. The water was pretty clean because it was a spring-fed lake, and the dock was in good shape. There was also a rope swing in front of the cottage and you could build up a little energy, swing out over the lake and drop in. It was great fun for the kids.

Pat and I bought a small sail boat, called a Sunfish, which we stored at the cottage. It was a simple fiberglass boat with one sail, but it was fun. You had to know the basics of sailing to use it, and fortunately I had done a little bit of sailing at the Clark Lake Yacht Club so I was able to handle it. We also got a car-top carrier for it and took it on several trips up to other lakes in Michigan.

When we were living in Pittsburgh, it was about a six-hour drive to the cottage and we went every summer. From Princeton, it was about twelve hours. The kids were older and liked to stay longer so several summers we met Pat's parents, Mickey and Charlie, early in the summer at a half-way place along Route 80 at Brookville, Pennsylvania, about six hours from each of us. They would go back with the kids to the cottage and we would make our drive there later in the summer when I took vacation time.

Even on home leaves from Europe, we would send the kids to the cottage. One time, when we were living in Paris, Pat's parents flew to Belgium where I picked them up at the Brussels airport. After traveling in Europe for a couple of weeks, they flew back to Detroit with the kids in tow. Pat and I then left on a month-long auto trip of Europe. After our vacation, I flew to Detroit to pick them up right in the middle of President Reagan's air controller strike. That time, they were at the cottage for over a month. They enjoyed going there very much, their grandparents loved having them there, and it became an important part of their lives for almost twenty years.

CHAPTER 45
Parents 50th/A Tribute to Gilbert

In July 1976 our parents were to celebrate their 50th wedding anniversary. The siblings and I decided that we wanted to have a surprise party for them followed by a family reunion. We first contacted First Methodist Church in Bowling Green and arranged to use the social hall as a place for the party. Then Pat and I did some research and found a suitable collection of seven guest cottages on Island Lake, on the opposite side of the lake from her parents cottage. This was a convenient location for the reunion, about an hour and a half north of the party location. Pat wrote up an invitation and we were good to go.

We developed a list of invitees after consulting with several of our parents' friends, but after the invitations were mailed, we heard from several people who had been left off of the list. It was not our intention to exclude anyone. But, by trying to keep it a secret from our parents, we made it difficult to develop a comprehensive list of everyone who might want to attend. We finally decided that we needed to consult with Lottie re the attendees and opened the party up to anyone who wanted to come. We had the relevant information promulgated in the church announcements.

The party was a great success. At least Gilbert appeared to be surprised. Many of Gilbert's faculty colleagues showed up along with a number of Mom's friends. Several of our former schoolteachers showed up as well. We had 50-60 people in all in addition to the family members.

And after the party the siblings and their families caravanned up to Island Lake for the reunion. Gilbert had been ailing and was not able to drive so one of the family members drove him and Mom up in their car. We had a fun time at the reunion and Gilbert especially enjoyed playing with his grandkids. We gathered in one of the cottages each night to sing songs and generally have a good time.

It was only a couple of weeks later that I was master of ceremonies for a Finance Industry sponsored customer executive conference we were holding at the facilities of the Woodrow Wilson School at Princeton University. There were about 300 customers in attendance. It was one of first events of this type that we had conducted. The facilities were very good since there was a large auditorium for the "main tent" and several smaller spaces for the breakout sessions.

We were in the middle of the second morning of the three-day conference when Ben Bruton, one of the other IBM managers, who was working on the conference, called me aside. He had a very somber look on his face. My father had passed away in his sleep the previous night. I was speechless. I had been with him just a few weeks earlier at the reunion. Fortunately, I had scripted the IBM portions of the conference. I gave Ben the control book, went home and made plans to go back to Bowling Green for the funeral.

I knew that Gilbert was not doing well health-wise. In the past years he had had a heart attack and several small strokes, and he had not been very active at the reunion. Apparently he had decided to hang on until the 50th anniversary party and the reunion and, according to our mother, the night before he passed away in his sleep, he told her that he had lived long enough.

He was 76 years old and had lived a full life. He was a husband, father, teacher, author, disciplinarian, mentor and example. He may have had his faults but he had many talents and he used them all. He did not waste them.

CHAPTER 46
The Selected International Account Program

We had a really top-flight group of managers in the Finance Industry when I was there, and several of them went on to very senior positions in IBM. I was beginning to realize that to get promoted from my job was going to be difficult, since those other managers were all probably ahead of me in the promotion queue.

When I first joined the IBM Finance Industry, one of the responsibilities that I inherited was the Selected International Account (SIA) Program that was sponsored by the World Trade Corporation. This was the program that supported large banking institutions like Citibank, Chase, Bankers Trust and Bank of America, that had international organizations with overseas branches. But it was one of those general programs that was not very important to the IBM Industry Director. He was more focused on the industry specific check processing and retail banking products in the US, and he wanted as little involvement with the SIA as possible.

What the program involved was a bit of people management (there were three people in New York City involved in the program), a bit of interface with the World Trade people in White Plains, New York and a bit of overseas travel. I would make probably two to three trips to Europe each year, normally to London or Paris, since most of the international banking activity at that time was in Europe. And I did not mind that at all. And possibly a trip to Mexico City as well to meet with the Latin and South American representatives. So I was the one manager in the finance industry who had direct contacts with the IBM World Trade organization.

In the spring of 1976, after we had started on the implementation of the industry product task force recommendations, I was asked to represent our director, John Bishop, at one of the meetings in White Plains of all of the industry directors. A representative of the EMEA (Europe/MiddleEast/Africa) organization was there and gave a presentation on the ongoing implementation of the industry centers in Europe. He was looking for experienced IBM managers to help staff these groups. He said that there were opportunities for US managers with industry center experience to help replicate what existed in the US organization into Europe.

Well, the first chance I got, I talked to John Bishop about the discussion and commented that I thought an assignment to World Trade might be a good step in my career. I think at the time, John thought that it would take me out of the main stream and might not be as good as some other options, but it was on the table.

Over the course of the next nine months I had several opportunities to visit Europe and, in particular, met with the Director of the IBM Finance Industry Center located outside of London. He was going to be replacing one or more of his managers in the next six months or so and said that I could be a good candidate. So we started a dialogue. But that director got replaced and I then had to then strike up a relationship with his successor, which I found the opportunity to do. So I was working on the situation, but having little success.

Then in January 1977 I had a scheduled SIA meeting in London. The day before I left on the trip John Bishop called me and told me to extend my trip to go to Amsterdam to visit the Scientific and Cross Industry Center (SCIC) which was located in Uithoorn, just south of Amsterdam. I arrived in Amsterdam's Schiphol Airport on a cold and dreary afternoon. The drive the next morning from my hotel to the industry center was along icy roads. I wondered what I was getting myself into.

When I got to the center, the Industry Director with whom I was supposed to meet was tied up in meetings. (It turned out he was being replaced.) And I was asked to meet with one of the Industry Managers, Jim Webster, instead. I found out that Jim was scheduled to return back to Canada sometime during the coming summer. The center was going to be taking on a new mission with a new text/office system being developed in England and Germany and a local Dutch manager had been identified to lead the team. But he did not have the Industry experience they wanted in the manager, and they were concerned about the success of the mission. They were now looking for someone who had industry staff experience. But since they were in the process of hiring a new director for the center at the same time, no decisions were going to be made for the near term.

I spent all of my time in a conference room and did not even get the chance to tour the center. The place was all kind of drab. It was interesting, but I did not get a good impression of the center, or my chances, and flew back to the states somewhat disappointed.

As I mentioned earlier, I had sung in the University of Michigan Men's Glee Club with the tenor Bob McGrath, who, after Michigan, joined PBS Television in a new program called Sesame Street. He was the "Bob" on Sesame Street for many years.

I had tracked him down and had asked him if my two children. Scott and Kelly, now ages seven and four could attend a filming of a Sesame Street show. He agreed and on a day in March 1977, we went up to the Sesame Street Studio on the upper West side of New York City to meet with Bob, and Bert & Ernie, and Big Bird and the whole gang. My kids sat right alongside the set and it was a memorable experience. Then Bob joined us for lunch. What a treat. We drove home feeling great and arrived shortly after dinner.

Just after we arrived at home the phone rang. It was John Bishop. I had just been offered a position as Industry Manager at the Scientific and Cross Industry Center in The Netherlands and needed to contact the International Assignment Office in White Plains to set up a look-see trip to Amsterdam. Two wonderful events in one day.

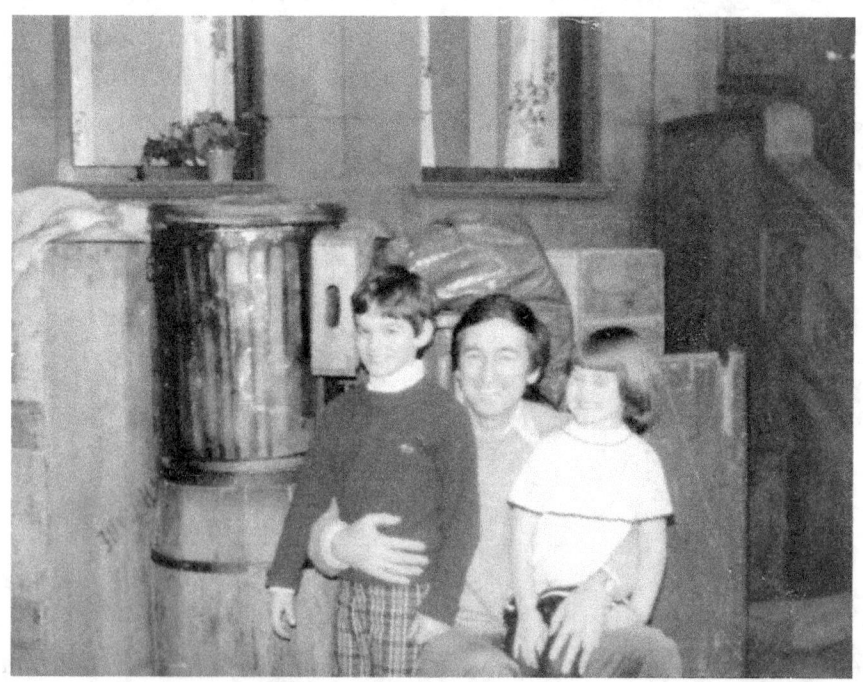

Scott and Kelly with Bob McGrath at Sesame Street- 1977

CHAPTER 47
Life in Wassenaar

Pat and I flew to Amsterdam in April 1977 for our look-see trip. The first couple of days did not go well at all. We did not see anything that would work for a family with two small children. The homes that they showed us were in busy sections of downtown Amsterdam, some of them where the furniture had to be hauled up on a hook from the outside of the house. We were quite discouraged.

Then I stopped by the office and ran into one of the US assignees, Jack Bazley, who would be working for me. He was assigned to a special project with Shell Oil Company in The Hague and suggested that we look in Wassenaar, a small Dutch town located between Leiden and The Hague, where a number of Americans were living. It also had some facilities of the American School of The Hague.

The IBM International Assignment Rep in Amsterdam had not told us anything about Wassenaar. But somehow we got the address of a real estate office there and drove down, not knowing what to expect. Well, we met the most delightful Dutch real estate lady and she just happened to have a side-by-side typical Dutch house that was going to be available in our time frame and in our price range. Bingo. We saw the house and were convinced. All she asked in return was that we bring her a case of Campbell's tomato soup in our boat shipment. We agreed and signed a two-year lease.

The house was located near the center of Wassenaar just down the street from the Molen (windmill) in the town and close to a number of the village shops, including the cheese shop, green grocer, butcher and the local branch of the Amro bank. Pat would be able to ride her bicycle to town to do the local shopping. It turned out to be an excellent choice for the kids as well since there was a movie theater that showed films in English on Saturday afternoon, within walking distance from our new home.

Life in Wassenaar was very pleasant. It was often called the "Golden Ghetto" because of the number of embassy homes in the community. There were a number of kids in town that went to the American School of The Hague, so our children had ample play-mates. And there were a number of US expats living in town as well as a number of Dutchmen married to American wives. So it was an enjoyable living experience. I used to tell people that the move from Princeton to Wassenaar had less culture shock than the move from Pittsburgh to Princeton. There was even a grocery store that special-ized in selling American products.

And the Dutch people loved the Americans. The neighbors were very friendly to us and the ones that lived during the Second World War remembered how the Americans helped overcome the problems of the German occupation, particularly the food shortages in the winter of 1944. They would invite us over for sherry in the afternoon and tell stories of the war. At night they would keep their front window curtains open while watching television. It was said that you could walk around the block in our community and keep up with a television show as you walked past the front windows of each house.

We had several vendors who delivered goods directly to our house including the "chicken" man who dropped off a package of chicken on most Sunday nights, even if we were out. And the milkman who would drop off a case of Heinekens if you preferred that in addition to your milk order. And the knife sharpener, etcetera. The list goes on.

I bought a Simca hatch-back car. We could put the kids in back with some children's books and they were content, so on the weekends we would take the Michelin guide and make drives around the country to check out the sights. When Scott was studying castles in school, we were able to make a weekend trip to the Mosel and Rhine rivers in Germany to visit a number of castles in person. It was really neat to be able to do that.

We were also a short distance from the university town of Leiden and also the town of Delft, known for the blue and white tiles and the painter Vermeer, and we enjoyed taking visitors to those places.

I won't go into all of the travels that we made from Holland, but we visited a large number of places, both by car and by plane, Michelin guide in hand. Belgium was just a short drive away. Kelly had a kindergarten class that made a ski trip to Germany and Scott's class had Thanksgiving week flights to London, so international travel was a normal part of life.

The Dutch were big travelers themselves dating back for hundreds of years, and the ones that we befriended were always telling us of the next place to visit. They were also great linguists and spoke multiple languages; they knew that most people would not learn Dutch and so they became fluent in many other languages, especially English. A Dutch girl, who lived across the street, was a frequent baby sitter and she spoke five languages.

We had also brought our cat, Angel, with us and the stories about her would fill another book.

So Holland was a very enjoyable living experience and an enjoyable travel experience as well..

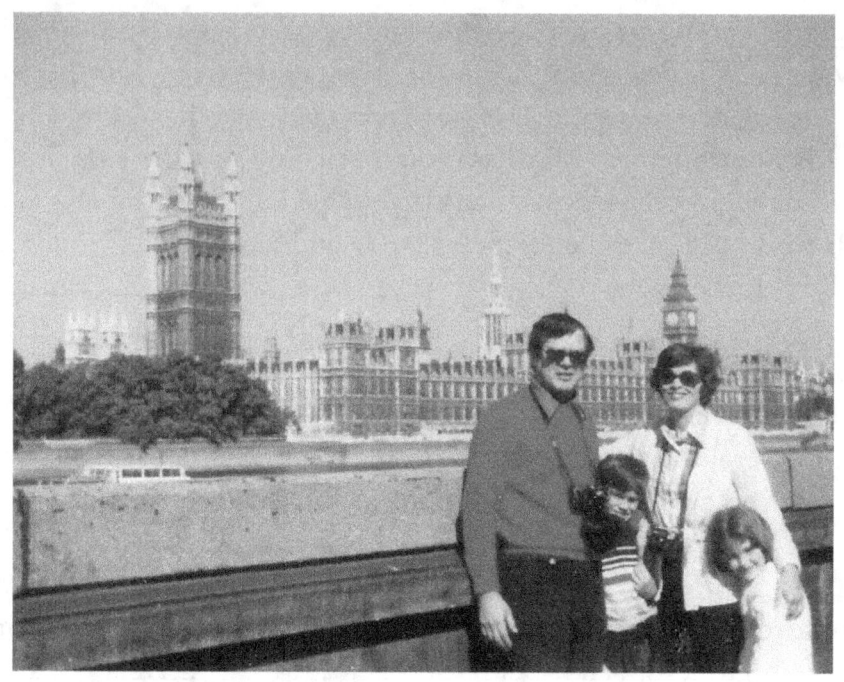

With Pat, Scott and Kelly in London

CHAPTER 48
Brigadier Doyle

Shortly after moving to Holland in May 1977, I had to go to the IBM facility in Hursley, England for a review meeting on the new office system product that was being developed there for which my team had the European marketing responsibility. Hursley was famous in England as the place for the design, development and manufacturing of the Spitfire aircraft that were so instrumental in the defense of London during the "Battle of Britain" in the Second World War. It had been taken over by IBM as a development lab sometime after the war.

This was a meeting of the IBM product managers from all of the major European countries as well as the US and was quite an important meeting for the upcoming announcement of the product across Europe. The Scientific and Cross Industry Center (SCIC) in Uithoorn, Netherlands had the European marketing mission for the product, and I was the responsible manager. It was also my first chance to meet many of the managers that I would be interfacing with during my assignment to SCIC.

After the meeting, we were scheduled to meet at a local inn called the Potters Heron for dinner and lodging. I stayed at the lab for a bit after the meeting to meet with the UK product development manager and then went by cab to the Potters Heron. When I arrived, I found that my room had been assigned to someone else in our group even though I had a guaranteed reservation. And since it was during the time of the Queen's fleet review taking place in nearby Portsmouth, the hotel was full and I had no place to stay.

I asked the hotel manager what he recommended that I do. He said that he had a friend, named Brigadier Doyle, who ran a guesthouse in the nearby New Forest and that he would call him. After a few minutes on the phone, he returned to tell me that he had arranged a room for me, that I should have dinner with the rest of the group and that he would arrange for a cab to take me to the guesthouse after dinner. So I felt better about the situation, although I was a little nervous about what I would find when I met up with Brigadier Doyle.

It was about two hours later that I showed up at the guesthouse, where I was met at the door by the brigadier. As you might imagine, he was a fairly heavyset elderly gentleman, well dressed and wearing a cravat. As I entered the door, he asked me if I would like a bit of sherry in the sitting room. I accepted the offer. I found out that he was a widower, that he and his wife had been operating the guesthouse together, and that after she passed away, he had decided to operate it by himself. He had about four to five guests each night, each in single rooms, mostly corporate customers.

Adjacent to the sitting room was a library. I asked if I could look around, and as I did so, holding my glass of sherry, I noticed a number of Sherlock Holmes books. I had been a fan of Sherlock Holmes for many years and was familiar with the titles. I opened up one of the books and noticed on the facing page, the inscription: "to my nephew, A. Conan Doyle." Another book had the same inscription. All of a sudden, my casual meeting with Brigadier Doyle had taken an ironic twist to it.

I asked the brigadier for more information. He acknowledged that he was indeed the nephew of A. Conan Doyle, the author of the Sherlock Holmes stories and had been raised by him. I told him that the inscribed books were probably extremely valuable and should not be left unlocked in the library. He was nonplused and could care less.

This was also the time when there were a number of "newly found manuscripts" of Sherlock Holmes that were appearing in the US press. I asked him if that was of any concern to him. He said that while he was the last living representative of the estate, he did not have time to get into any issues with the manuscripts, and instead wanted to know at what time I wanted my English breakfast delivered to my room in the morning. I went to bed amazed. Here was an individual sitting on possibly a fortune in books, more concerned only about breakfast for one of his customers.

The next morning at the designated time, there was a tap on my door and my breakfast was delivered, complete with eggs and strawberry jam. After that, a cab appeared at the designated time to take me to the Hursley site. I told my colleagues, who had stayed at the Potters Heron, "You will not believe what happened to me last night." And I went on to explain my surprising evening with Brigadier Doyle.

I had many other opportunities to stay at the Potters Heron during the course of my years working in Europe, but none matched my experience with staying with Brigadier Doyle in the New Forest. I have the bill from that lodging somewhere in my "stuff." And I am still a big fan of Sherlock Holmes, particularly his "turn for both observation and deduction." AKA "varking."

CHAPTER 49
We Move to Paris

My assignment to the IBM Scientific and Cross Industry Center (SCIC) in The Netherlands, was originally to be for three years. But in the spring of 1979 after about two years, the decision was made to close the center and combine it with another center that already existed in Paris.

John Bishop had gotten the international bug, and had moved to Paris after the first of the year to take over the executive responsibility for Industry Marketing in Europe. Shortly after he and his family had arrived, we invited them to visit us in Holland. They drove up and we had a nice weekend together and showed them a number of our favorite spots in Amsterdam and the Wassenaar area. At the end of our visit, he said that there might be a job for me in Paris in the restructured Industry Center organization.

The lease that we had signed on our home was for two years although we had hoped to be able to extend it. But in May 1979 a nice looking Dutchman showed up at the front door with a bouquet of flowers. He said that he was the owner, was back in the country, and wanted to move back into his house. But he was nice enough to allow us to stay until we found other quarters.

At the time, the IBM people working in Paris thought that Paris was the end all. Why would anyone want to work or live anywhere else? Well, we were happy at the time living and working in Holland. My team had received an IBM Outstanding Contribution award for the work that we had done in announcing and supporting the new product across Europe, so I was well thought of in the IBM community. Besides, the Dutch were very nice. We had visited Paris and had not heard such pleasant things about the French. But with the return of the landlord, and SCIC closing down sometime in the future, a move to Paris was an option that we needed to consider. And as with anything else, it needed to be approved by IBM.

Things started moving forward in the summer, when John invited Pat and me for a look-see trip to Paris. We took the bateau mouche dinner cruise, talked to some IBM friends who were living in Paris about the housing, schools, etcetera and John asked if we wanted him to move forward with the approvals. Pat and I discussed it, and said yes.

It took several more months, however, to get my assignment to Paris approved. It was for an additional two and a half years until June 1982. We were able to negotiate a six-month extension of our lease in Wassenaar, and in November 1979 we moved into our new digs at Une Place Santos Dumont, Saint Cloud, France. It was a residential area named after the French aviator, and the house and square had been featured on an out-of-print French post card.

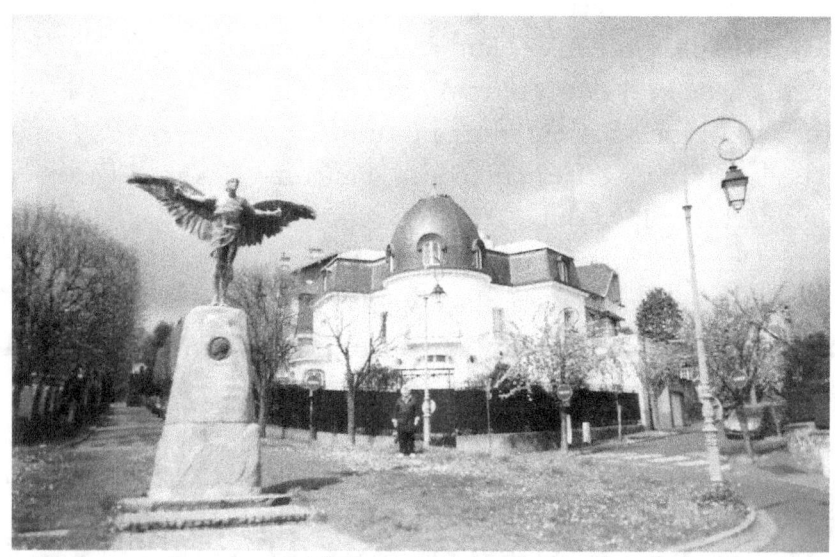

Une Place Santos Dumont

CHAPTER 50
Une Place Santos Dumont

Life in Paris was quite a bit different from life in Holland. We had lived in Europe for two and a half years and considered ourselves experienced expats. But Paris was a different experience. For one thing, the shopkeepers and people that Pat had to deal with on a daily basis usually did not speak English. You had to speak French to communicate or else have a friend who did. So daily living was much more complicated.

On the other hand, the museums and restaurants in Paris were world class. Not that Holland did not have great museums. The Rijksmuseum in Amsterdam, for example, is a great museum. But Paris had world-class museums in abundance. And there was an art teacher at the American School of Paris who scheduled frequent Saturday morning lectures at the Louvre, the Cluny or other various museums. I think that the Cluny was one of my favorites. And, of course, there is not much to compare between Dutch cooking and French cooking. One of the great pleasures of Paris was getting out the Michelin guide and picking out the next great restaurant that you could talk to your friends about.

The IBM visiting "dignitaries" frequented Paris; they rarely frequented Amsterdam. So I would have people visiting Europe for some valid reason and then contacting me to advise that they would be in Paris at such and such a time and wanted to know if we could get together. Some of the wives tried to specialize in French cooking at home, but most just went the restaurant route instead. So we developed a list of favorites.

Our home in Wassenaar had been a delight. We had few problems, and the kids enjoyed living there. Our home in Saint Cloud was another story. It was a large three-story house that had a separate apartment on the third floor. When we moved in, the third floor was occupied by a US-French couple with the wife from the states. She was a good resource for us, and very helpful in knowing the immediate area.

The house was conveniently located. There was a train station in front of the house that made a leisurely trip to the Left Bank. Another train station up the hill in back of the house made a quick trip to La Defense, where my office was located, and then to St. Lazare Train Station in downtown Paris. From the front veranda you had an excellent view of the Tour Eiffel and the Bois de Boulogne and from the deck, off of Scott's bedroom, you could see the Arc de Triumph. So it was an excellent location.

But after a year the American tenant upstairs moved out and a pure French family moved in. Not so good. We also had problems with the house; the furnace, the wiring, etcetera. And the landlord lived in Toulouse and was not helpful in resolving our problems. We also found out that the area where we lived was considered good pickings for robberies. A number of homes in the area were pilfered at different times, including the homes of some of our American friends. We became very sensitive to not being one of the unlucky ones. We once experienced a robbery actually taking place at one of the homes across the street from us. We called the police, but they did not appear to be in any hurry to show up. I saw one of the thieves drop down from the second story and figured he must have broken a leg or something. I went down into the street with a baseball bat, but the thieves got away. The police arrived about twenty minutes later.

We also had an interesting time with French customs. Pat had purchased a US spec Volkswagen Rabbit while in Holland. For French customs, it was a big problem. The car id number was in the wrong place, the head-lights were wrong, and the side-lights were not allowed. I don't think that they liked anything about the car. I was travelling a lot and did not have a lot of time to devote to the problems. It took the better part of a year before we got the car approved for French plates by French customs. And Pat and I celebrated the event with a glass of French champagne.

But, if you could overlook living with the Parisians, life in Paris was not so bad. I had an interesting job and traveled throughout Europe on a weekly basis. We met a number of interesting people, through IBM, The American Church of Paris, and the American School of Paris. And our kids made some good friends at school as well.

We enjoyed travelling on the weekends, much of it with the kids. The Normandy Beaches, Honfleur and the Loire Valley were just a couple of hours away and provided interesting spots to visit. We found a favorite chateau in the Loire Valley close to Chenonceaux that had a tower room where the four of us could all sleep. Chartres and Versailles were about an hour away. There was much to do on the weekends. You could drive to Switzerland in five hours, Belgium in two, and Germany in six. We were centrally located to travel, and close to many different wine areas. As John Bishop liked to say "When you first arrive in France, you spend three hours visiting the chateau and one hour at the restaurant. After you have been here a while, you spend one hour visiting the chateau, and three hours at the restaurant."

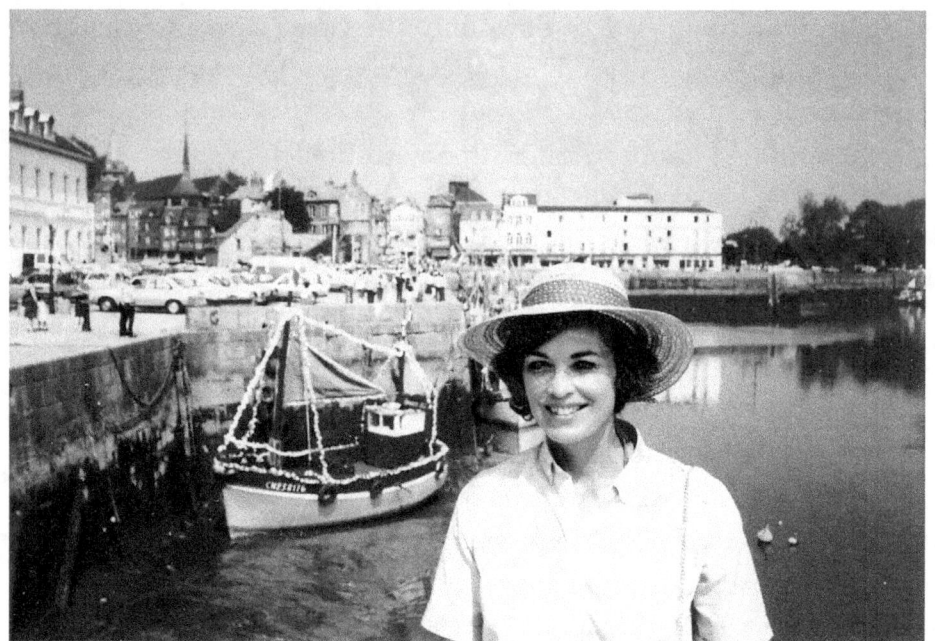

Pat at Honfleur, France-1981

And travel we did. I won't go into all of the places that we visited, either Pat & I on a business trip, or the four of us with the kids in tow, either by car or by plane. I will just share one such experience.

I was responsible for the team marketing a new office system product. It had a lot of European involvement since the hardware had been developed in Hursley, England, and the software in Sindelfingen, Germany. We had developed a lot of deliverables for the product, including a movie, slide sets, foil presentations, etcetera. And because it was new and a cross industry product, a lot of the industry managers wanted me or one of my team to present at meetings that they might be holding, particularly customer executive sessions. It demonstrated that IBM was investing in new markets.

I was invited to go to one such customer executive meeting in the south of France. I had not checked out the details of the place in advance since Pat and I were going to take a couple of days for vacation in Cannes prior to the meeting. I had rented a car and on the day we were due to check in, and we arrived mid afternoon, hot and sweaty after a couple-hour car ride. Our IBM host met us and invited us to join the party for a buffet that they were having. I felt a little uncomfortable since I had not known that they were going to have the buffet and we did not have time to clean up before eating. But we joined them and had excellent food. And then we saw our room, overlooking the grounds that overlooked the Mediterranean. Wonderful as well.

The place that we were staying was called Hotel du Cap Eden Roc located on Cap D'Antibes. It is one of the most exclusive hotels in the south of France, if not all of Europe, and is included in the book of 1000 places to see before you die. If I had been smart and checked it out more in advance, I would have made sure we arrived in time to get cleaned up and would also have arranged my schedule to take advantage of the IBM host's offer to stay on a few more days at his expense. As it was, at least I gave them a good presentation and used all of the tools of the trade that I had brought with me. And they appreciated that.

IBM EMEA was responsible for the countries in Europe, the Middle East and Africa. But our primary focus was on the four majors; United Kingdom, Germany, France and Italy. The next tier included The Netherlands, Belgium, Switzerland and Spain. And then there were the rest. South Africa was too far away to be of much interest and reps from EMEA rarely went there. It was easier to travel to the countries that made the most difference to the bottom line of the product or marketing program for which you were responsible.

The Industry Centers were spread out over the various countries; Finance Center in London, Manufacturing and Process Centers in Germany, Public Sector in Rome, Distribution Industry Center in Paris, and, until it was closing down, Scientific and Cross Industry

Center in The Netherlands. So travel in the course of doing your job could take you almost anywhere in Europe.

Over the two and a half years in Paris, I was invited to participate in a large number of meetings throughout Europe, both IBM internal and customer executive sessions, and visited many of the historic towns and cities. The one thing that I did not do was to over-extend my welcome at any of these meetings on the expense account of the host. There were several SCIC staff members who got a reputation for showing up uninvited at meetings at exotic locations at IBM expense. None of them ever worked for me and I usually stayed just long enough to fulfill the responsibilities for which I was invited.

But over our five years in Europe, Pat and I probably visited every major city in Western Europe at one time or another. Our favorite cities were probably Florence, Italy, and Munich, Germany. We also had opportunities to travel with other groups and had visited Russia, the Greek Islands, the Algarve in Portugal, and Egypt on those trips. I found the tour to Egypt as probably the most interesting with visits to the pyramids, the Valley of the Kings and Abu Simbel. I believe that Pat preferred Cannes and the south of France.

―――――――――――

In April 1982 I received a call on a Friday afternoon from the states, from Clark Grimes, an IBMer that I had worked with in the Finance Industry in 1974 and 1975. He had moved through the ranks and was now the Director of Finance Industry Marketing in Princeton, having replaced John Bishop. He had a job opening in his organization for a second level manager and offered me the job. He wanted a response by Monday. I had several other options in play but none that were as good and all involved moves to either White Plains, New York, or the Washington, DC area.

I discussed the call with Pat and then called Clark back and accepted the job.

CHAPTER 51
La Rentrée

Paris closes down in the month of August and almost everyone goes on vacation. The restaurants are closed, shops are closed. The city shuts down. Then in September, everyone returns. It is called la rentrée. And everything picks up again.

Our rentrée to the States took place not in September but in June 1982. After five years in Europe it was a major event in our lives. We were moving back into the same house that we had purchased in 1974 and rented out during our time in Europe. We had been back to Princeton a couple of times on home leave in the previous five years, but I was a little nervous about getting back into the swing of things in the Finance Industry. In Europe, you had quite a bit of freedom in what you did since there was not a huge infrastructure in the organization. In the US, you had a hierarchical organization with a lot of senior people who knew a little bit about what you were doing and just might want to put their two cents in. So it was a different kind of structure.

They also wanted me to start right away. So I started flying back to the states in April 1982 to attend meetings and get oriented. Along the way, Clark Grimes got promoted again so I was dealing with a new Industry Director, Peter Dance, who did not know me at all. Finally, the end of June, we took our last family European vacation, in Cannes, and flew back to the states. I immediately took off

for Los Angeles and other destinations and left Pat to fend for herself
for a while in the local hotel. Finally, the boat with our household
goods arrived, and we were able to get settled in our house again. The
kids were now 12 and 9. They renewed old friendships and settled
back into the Princeton school system. We were home again for what
we hoped would be a long time.

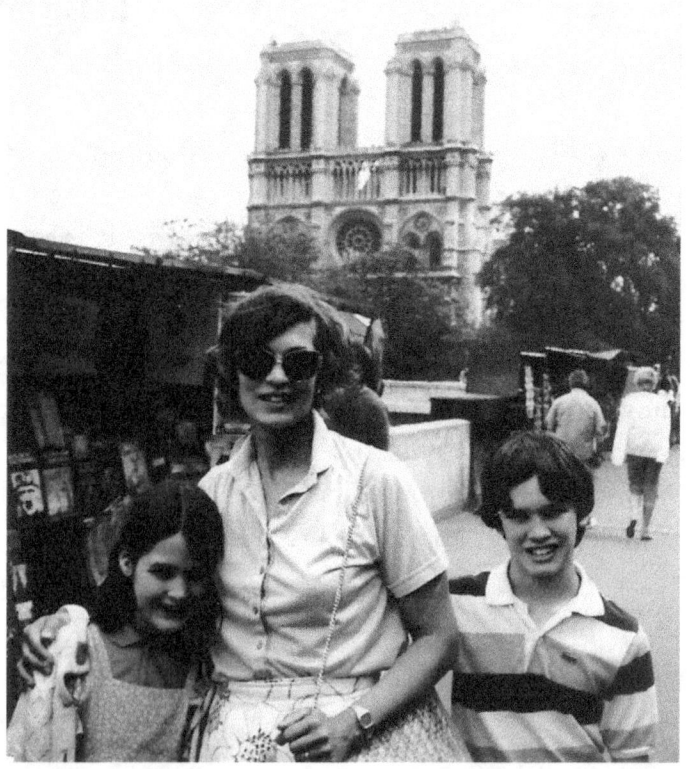

"Pat with Scott and Kelly at Notre Dame" -1982

CHAPTER 52
Lottie, part 2

After my father, Gilbert passed away in 1976, my mother, Lottie, stayed busy with her crafts. She had even traveled to visit us in Holland. After a week there my whole family flew with her to London, where we enjoyed another few days before we put her on a plane back to the US.

In the early 1980s, she had started to get letters from the Bowling Green State University development office and didn't know what to do about them. She brought them to my attention one summer when I was on a home leave from Paris. I contacted the university to find out what it was all about and learned that they were interested in raising money by focusing on endowments for a few of the retired or deceased professors. Gilbert was one of the candidates.

I talked to Mom about it and we agreed that, after I returned from my assignment in Paris and had more time to devote to it, we would meet with the university to discuss it. So in the summer of 1982, after my return from Paris, we met not just with the development office, but also with the dean of the School of Business Administration. Everyone supported the endeavor. This led to writing letters to many of Dad's former students and also his faculty colleagues; and eventually to the establishment of the Gilbert Cooke Memorial Scholarship Fund.

After Lottie passed away in 1996, it became the Gilbert and Lottie Cooke Memorial Scholarship Fund. With the help of contributions from my siblings, and the support of the Business School in contacting former students, it is now the largest non-corporate scholarship in the business school.

While Mom was alive, my brother, Dean and my sister, Janet and I tried to make sure that Mom was able to attend the annual scholarship presentations at BGSU where the recipients were honored. She enjoyed meeting with the university representatives as well as with the recipients of the awards. It was very satisfying to talk to the recipients as they were all very appreciative of having received the scholarship and, in some cases, could not have attended the university without it.

CHAPTER 53
The False Alarm

It is a week before Christmas 1983 about 6:30 in the evening and a group of us are hard at work at the IBM Finance Industry offices in Princeton. Peter Dance, the new director, is having a meeting of the product mangers down the hall and I am in my office trying to wrap things up for the day. All of a sudden I start to feel very weak and begin to slide down under my desk. I get up enough energy to get down the hallway and ask Brian Warman to come out of the meeting. I tell him that I am not feeling well and ask him if he could stay with me in my office for a bit. He agrees and he goes back with me to sit down.

Brian is a good friend and one of the first people that I met when I first came out to the industry in 1973. He was also helpful on my return from Paris the previous year.

After sitting in my office for a few minutes I told Brian that I was not feeling any better and ask him to call the rescue squad. He jokingly comments that he has had CPR training and could help me if I wanted him to. I thank him for his efforts and ask him to make the call.

Well, the rescue squad arrives within minutes with the stretcher, oxygen et al and I am shortly on my way to the emergency room at the Medical Center at Princeton. Brian calls my wife, Pat, to meet us there.

At the emergency room I am diagnosed as having had a heart attack and treated in that manner. I remember being asked about chest pain and said that I did have pain in my lower chest that was at a level of about 5 out of 10. It was not until about 24 hours later when things really started to change.

The pain started to move from my chest to my lower abdomen. When I was asked again about the pain level I said that it was about a 9 moving to a 10. The nurses conducted some new tests. My wife had been with me for a long while but had gone home to care for our children. She was called by our surgeon friend, Dr. Jay Chandler, to come to the hospital but was not told why.

When Pat got to the hospital she was told that I did not have a heart attack at all but had had a ruptured appendix. I was going to undergo emergency surgery. As I was being rolled into the surgical suite starting to go under from the anesthesia I remember looking up at Dr. Chandler and saying "We have got to stop meeting like this." And then I went under.

The operation was a success. I had indeed had a ruptured appendix and had severe infection called peritonitis in my stomach area so they could not sew me up but had to put in a drain in the incision. The original pain in my chest was caused by my appendix rupturing in an upward position and then as that subsided, the pain moved to the original spot of my appendix in my abdomen.

But I was now in the hospital, Christmas was a week away and my stomach was really sore. One of the nurses made me a hug-me pillow that I could hold to my chest whenever I had to cough or laugh. My daughter, Kelly, brought a small artificial Christmas tree into my room to spruce it up. I remember that my roommate was a heart attack patient, and I thought, well when I get out of here, I will be ok but he will still have to deal with the after effects of the heart attack. I also thought about the hole in the ground in our backyard where we had a partially finished swimming pool due for completion in the spring and wondering whether I would ever be able to use it. And every morning one of Dr. Chandler's associates would come in about 7AM and pull the drain in my abdomen out a little further.

I started asking Dr. Chandler about how soon I could get out of the hospital and he said that it all depended on how soon my infection cleared up. Brian, Peter Dance and some of my other Finance Industry colleagues came over to see me and I was able to meet them out in a reception area. They started telling stories and jokes and I started laughing. Fortunately I had the hug-me pillow with me during this get together.

Finally my infection cleared up, the remainder of the drain in my stomach was pulled out and I was released from the hospital on the day before Christmas. The next day was a wonderful Christmas with my family, and I was on the road to recovery.

In a follow-up visit with Dr. Chandler, I inquired about a warm spot that I might visit to speed up my recovery. He said "Antigua." I had never been there and had never thought about going there, but on his suggestion I tucked it away for future consideration. And a month or so later, that is where Pat and I went to enjoy the sun and the beaches.

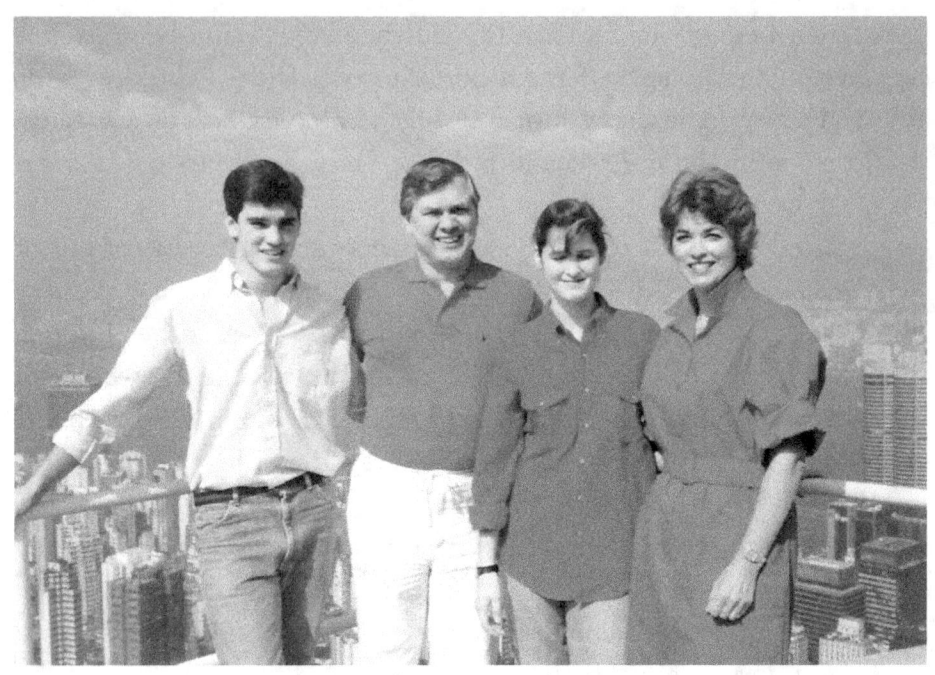

Cooke Family in Hong Kong - 1986

CHAPTER 54
"Dragon" Hamm

After recovering from my ruptured appendix surgery, for the next year or so things seemed to get back to normal. We used some of the money that we had saved in Europe to put a screened-in porch on the house, build a deck, and finish the swimming pool. I went through three more industry directors. And it started to become apparent that they wanted me to move on to another position, possibly a branch location manager. Scott by this time had settled in to the high school and had mentally charted out his courses for the next three years.

We were not sure how to respond to the discussions on moving. They had even asked me to meet with some executives of an IBM joint venture in White Plains. But then fate intervened again with another overseas opportunity.

John Bishop had come by Princeton in 1984 to let us know that he was taking a job as the country manager in South Korea and to ask if I was interested in going there. I was just recovering from my appendix surgery so I respectfully declined. But then in the spring of 1985 things changed again. Drayton Hamm was one of the managers that I had worked with in my early days in Finance Industry in 1974. I had lost track of where he was working, but he was in town for a few days and asked if he could stop by our house. We had not seen him for a while so we asked him to come to dinner. The three of us, Pat, Drayton and I sat together in our dining room.

He told us that he was working in Hong Kong as Finance Industry Manager in the South East Asia Region called SEAR. It was a small staff and supported Hong Kong, Taiwan, South Korea and the five ASEAN (Association of South East Asian Nations) countries; Indonesia, Malaysia, The Philippines, Singapore and Thailand, all places that I had never visited before. He was the only person supporting the Finance Industry. There were other staff members supporting other industries such as Manufacturing, Public Sector, Distribution, Process, etcetera. He was on a three-year assignment due to end the summer of 1986 and was responsible to find his own replacement.

He knew that I had been successful in the IBM Europe/Middle East/Africa (EMEA) organization and was interested in knowing if I might want to be his replacement. He said that the job was very comprehensive and covered all aspects of the Industry, from coordinating strategy, developing specific country operating plans, to customer calls, trouble shooting and coordinating visits from industry specialists from the US Finance Industry organization. He felt that I was well qualified for the position. He did not need to know right away but would probably need to know my intentions by later in the year.

After he left, Pat and I talked about it. I had not given a lot of thought to another overseas assignment, but given that we had never been to Asia and that the Industry was talking about me getting another position anyway, we decided to cash in some United Airlines mileage points and fly to Hong Kong to take a look. Pat's mother agreed to stay with the kids, and in August of 1985 we were off on the long plane trip to Asia.

Drayton arranged our hotel accommodations at the Hong Kong Shangri-la Hotel and set up a meeting with his management. He was an enthusiastic host and showed us many of his local shops, restaurants and haunts, including his Hong Kong tailor, Nelson David and Henry Ho, the shop where he bought his knock-off polo shirts. We learned that he had the local nickname "Dragon Hamm" based on his enjoyment of the area. The Shangri-La Hotel, where we were staying, was a very nice hotel on the Hong Kong harbor, and we made a weekend jaunt into Macau and mainland China and had a wonderful time. We were hooked. Now we had to convince our kids.

Kelly was the easiest. She had spent over half of her life living overseas and was up for anything international. Scott was the most difficult. He would be entering his junior year in high school if we moved again and had organized all of the courses he planned to take for the next two years. We didn't push him but over time he agreed to go. We contacted Drayton with our intentions, and shortly after the first of the year in 1986 the assignment was approved, and we were on our way with the "formal" look-see trip.

We found an apartment in the same building where Drayton lived on Old Peak Road. It was in what was called Mid-Levels about half way up the peak on the Hong Kong side. (The other side across the harbor was called the Kowloon side.) The apartment had four bedrooms and a separate amah quarters for a live-in maid, which we eventually had. We could walk to the central part of Hong Kong where the IBM offices were, although to get home one would probably want to take a taxi since it was uphill all the way.

We visited the Hong Kong International School (HKIS) where the kids would be going to school. We found out that there were a number of kids in the mid level apartments nearby who took the bus to the school; and the bus stopped just down the street from the apartment. It could not have been more convenient.

It turned out that Drayton had a job offer with IBM in NYC and took off as soon as my three-year assignment was announced. And so the end of April 1986, I started commuting from Princeton to Hong Kong, staying for three weeks each time followed up by a week in Princeton. We finally packed up our stuff into three piles, (air shipment, boat shipment and storage), and made the big move at the end of June stopping in Detroit where Pat's mom, Mickey, had organized a family going away party for us. And then we visited one of Pat's high school friends in Hawaii along the way.

Covering the territory and vacation/weekend traveling were a bit different in Asia than they had been in Europe. You could not drive or take the train anywhere, except the boat to Macau. You had to fly. But my territory was interesting, originally eight countries, Korea, Taiwan, Hong Kong and the five ASEANS; Indonesia, Malaysia, the Philippines, Singapore and Thailand; it eventually grew to include China, Australia and New Zealand.

I was on a plane about half the time, mostly flying Cathay Pacific, an excellent airline. I didn't go to China a lot but had several trips to Beijing and on one was able to bring Pat along to visit the Great Wall. I probably visited Bangkok, Thailand the most, since there was a marketing center there for which I had coordinating responsibility. Pat went with me a number of times and found the Shangri-la Hotel in Bangkok to be one of her favorites. It was located right along the river and, while it would take me a little longer to get to the office than from one of the downtown hotels, was well worth the extra time. And I used Saturday morning at the office in Hong Kong to get caught up on paperwork.

Many of the expats had live-in Filipino amahs and most of the apartments had maid's quarters so it was a ready-made situation. The amahs would cook, clean and also mastered the small Chinese washing machines. We did succumb to getting an amah as well, but held off for about a year before giving in, primarily because of the amount of laundry that our kids were generating. The amahs were also most helpful if you had some visiting "dignitaries" who wanted to see what dinner in a Hong Kong apartment was like. Our amah was a Filipino college grad named De Ling, but she could make more money working for us as a maid in Hong Kong and sending a portion home to her family in the Philippines.

Many of us were able to get corporate memberships at the American Club which was located a couple of buildings over from the IBM office. It was a nice life. And many of the expats were double dippers, who had already been on assignments in Europe and were experienced travelers. They were excellent sources of information.

Home leaves from Hong Kong were pretty neat. We could decide which way we wanted to travel around the globe, east or west. We had two home leaves during our three-year assignment. One year we went to Paris and Holland on the way home and then stopped in Malaysia on the way back. The next year we went on safari in Kenya and then to London on the way home and stopped in Hawaii on the way back. Not bad duty.

The safari was probably one of the best family vacations that we have ever had. One of the places where we stayed, "The Ark," was an ark-like structure built over a water hole that would house about 100 guests in ship-board-like cabins. A variety of animals would come to the water hole, and the Ark had various spots where one could view the animals. The animals came generally at night and if there was a new species that had not been seen that day, they would ring up your room to let you know. Pat and I chose to silence the alarm in our cabin. Kelly chose to be awakened.

When we met Kelly for breakfast the next morning, she said that she had been awakened to see new animals several times during the night. But more interesting was that many of the people joining her in the viewing station at the water hole were from Toledo, Ohio. We found out that about two-thirds of the guests staying at the Ark in the middle of Kenya that evening were on a tour from the Toledo Zoo. Small world.

I had hoped to be able to extend my assignment until the end of 1989 so Kelly could graduate from HKIS. But in 1988, IBM had a special program in effect to encourage people to take early retirement. I was eligible for the program, and in order to take advantage of it,

I had to start retirement in June 1989, earlier that I had planned. But we were still able to make arrangements for Kelly to graduate from HKIS the following June, after spending a semester at Princeton High School.

During my Hong Kong assignment, I was able to provide several people with the opportunity that Drayton Hamm had provided to me. I hired Jim Riemann from IBM in Charlotte to head up the banking center in Bangkok, and then identified Will Lowrimore as his replacement when Jim's assignment came to an end in 1988. At the end of my tour, I identified Jon Varvel, also from Charlotte, to replace me in Hong Kong. Interestingly enough, a year after Jon arrived in Hong Kong, IBM reorganized again and Jon ended up his tour in Japan. I have spoken to each of them since their return and they all have indicated that these tours in Asia were among the highlights of their IBM careers. So I was able to help pay back for some of the support that I had been given over the years.

All good things come to an end and ours ended with a funeral. Pat's mother had been diagnosed with brain cancer soon after we arrived in Hong Kong. She had put up a good fight for three years, but the month we were due to depart from Hong Kong, June 1989, she passed away, and Pat and I delayed our departure to go back to Detroit for the funeral. We had left a neighbor to look after our children when we were gone.

Much to our surprise when we turned on the television at our hotel in Detroit, they were showing pictures of the tanks in Tiananmen Square in Beijing. It was the week of the riots and there were also demonstrations in Hong Kong. We were worried about our kids, but knew that they were in good hands. We then returned to Hong Kong, moved into the Mandarin Hotel (one of Hong Kong's finest) while our household goods were being packed up and flew back to Princeton, stopping by Hawaii for a little R & R on the way back.

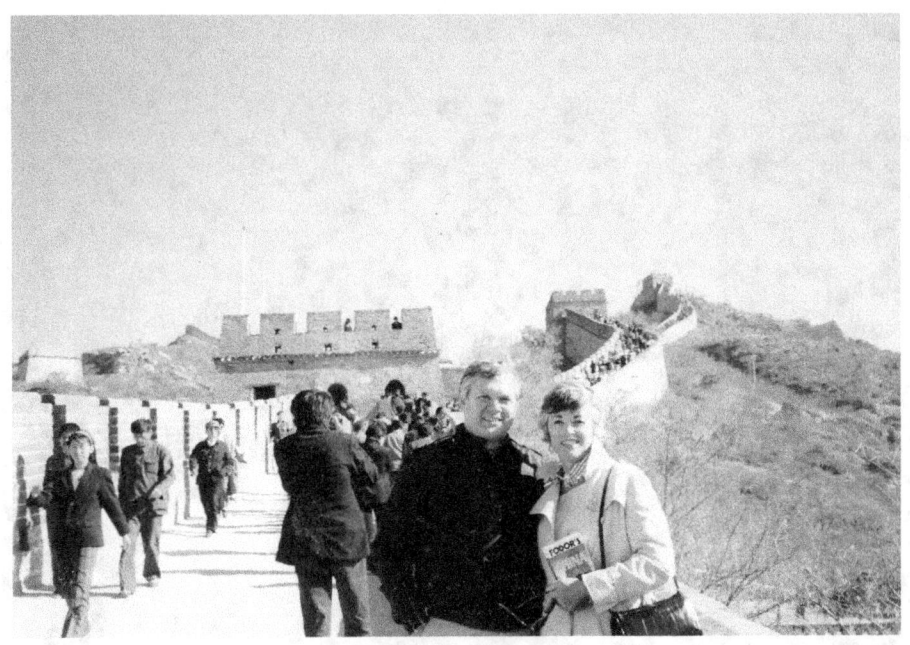

With Pat at the Great Wall of China-1988

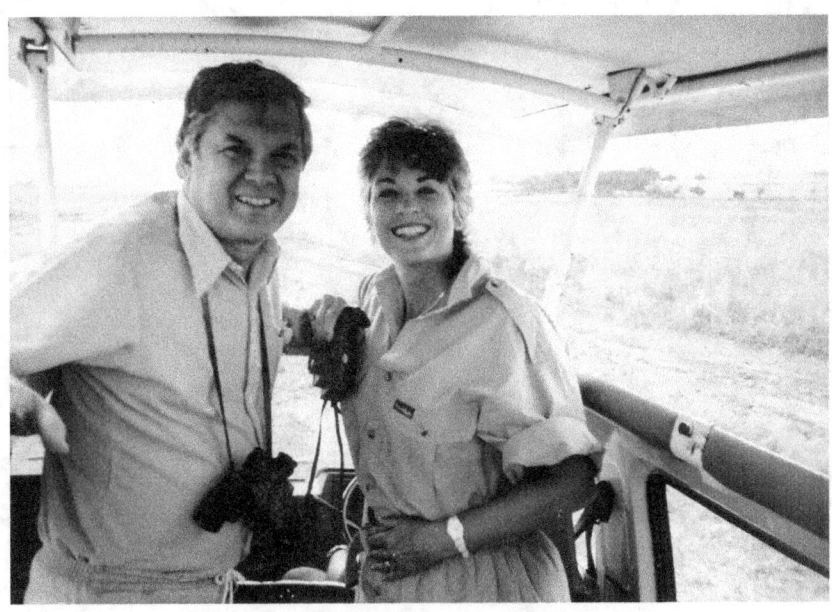

With Pat on Safari in Kenya-1988

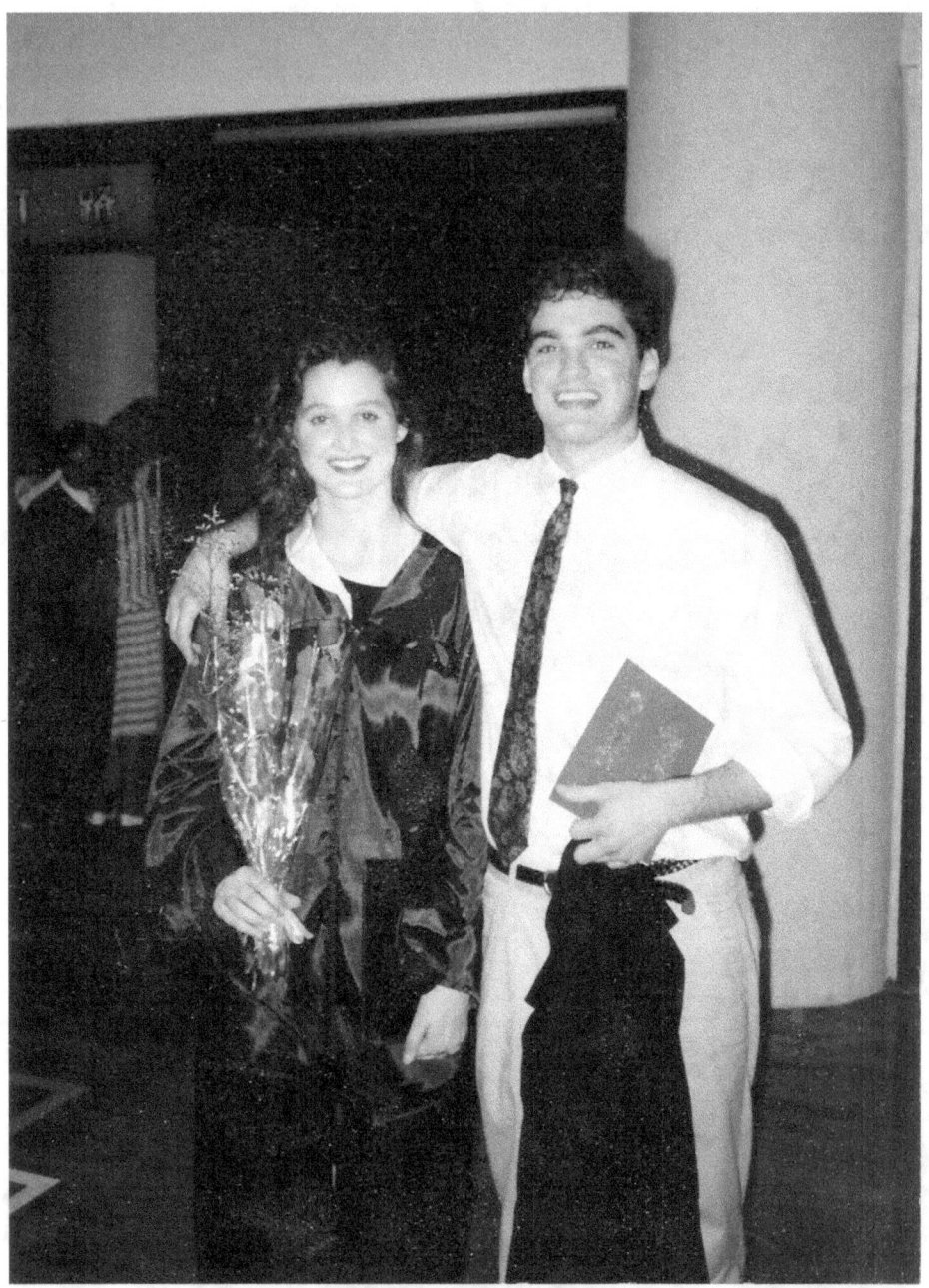

Scott and Kelly at Kelly's HKIS graduation-1990

CHAPTER 55
Three Different Cultures

In my thirty year career in IBM, I was fortunate to have spent eight years overseas in three excellent locations and had management positions on three continents; America, Europe and Asia. All three overseas locations involved different cultures but all were equally exciting.

Pat is frequently asked which of the three locations she liked the best. And she would reply that they were all the best in their own way. For Holland, it was a nice location for a growing family. For Paris, it was the ambiance, the restaurants and the museums. And for Hong Kong, it was the mixture of a New York City and a San Francisco with a pulse and excitement that was unmatched.

The social activities in the three locations were different as well. Holland did not have a lot of expats, but the ones there mostly lived in single-family homes or side-by-side duplexes, and a number in corporate-owned houses. Most tried to live close to the American School of The Hague, as we did. It was the only American school in Holland that had 12 grades. So a lot of the social activities of the community were focused on events at the school. There were other activities centered on the American Church of The Hague, a non-denominational church, and the American Baseball League, which sponsored games for the expat kids from T-ball on up and had a big 4th of July party each year. Add in a few dinner/bridge parties and you had it.

In Paris, the expats were scattered all around the city, many in single-family homes. The American School of Paris was near our house, but it did not seem to have the same dynamics in the community as the school did in The Hague. There was more in home entertaining for the expat wives to show off their new-found French cooking skills (Pat had gone to a week-long school in Chinon, a town along the Loire Valley famous for Jean D'Arc), and more just going out to the various restaurants in the city. One of our fondest memories was a New Year's Eve party in 1980 at John and Dianne Bishop's apartment on L' Avenue de la Bourdonnais in central Paris. There were five couples altogether and everyone brought something. One of the men had a French wife who taught us to sing La Marseillaise. And at midnight, we serenaded everyone in the street from the balcony with a toast of French champagne and the French national anthem.

IBM EHQ and the American Women's Club would normally throw one or two big bashes during the course of the year as well. The Women's Club party at Versailles was most memorable. The American Church of Paris was also a comforting presence and Tom Duggan, the minister there while we were in Paris, had previously served at our church in The Hague so we knew him well.

In Hong Kong almost everybody lived in high-rise apartments, most of them on Hong Kong Island, where you would have a walk or taxi ride to work. A few lived in single family homes or low-rise dwellings on the opposite side of the Island, but they had to balance their more traditional American-style housing with a longer commute. There were a number of dinner/bridge parties since many people had amahs that would take care of the cooking chores. But, on many weekends people would want to get out and about, to get away from the cramped- in feeling of the apartments. So there were junk rides to Lamma Island, parties at the American Club, or perhaps just hiking trips up to the peak or around the mid-levels of the island. And IBM would have its share of annual bashes as well.

I think for our children, of the three locations, Hong Kong was the best. They made friendships that they cherish to this day. They got excellent educations, and our daughter developed a love of Mandarin that she parlayed into a Georgetown University degree. They learned to enjoy junk cruises to the neighboring islands. And they found out that there was no legal drinking age at the various establishments in Hong Kong.

In our years of international living, we had experienced more than our fair share of international travel and good living. But Pat and I knew that on our return to Princeton in 1989, those days were going to be over: it was the end of an era.

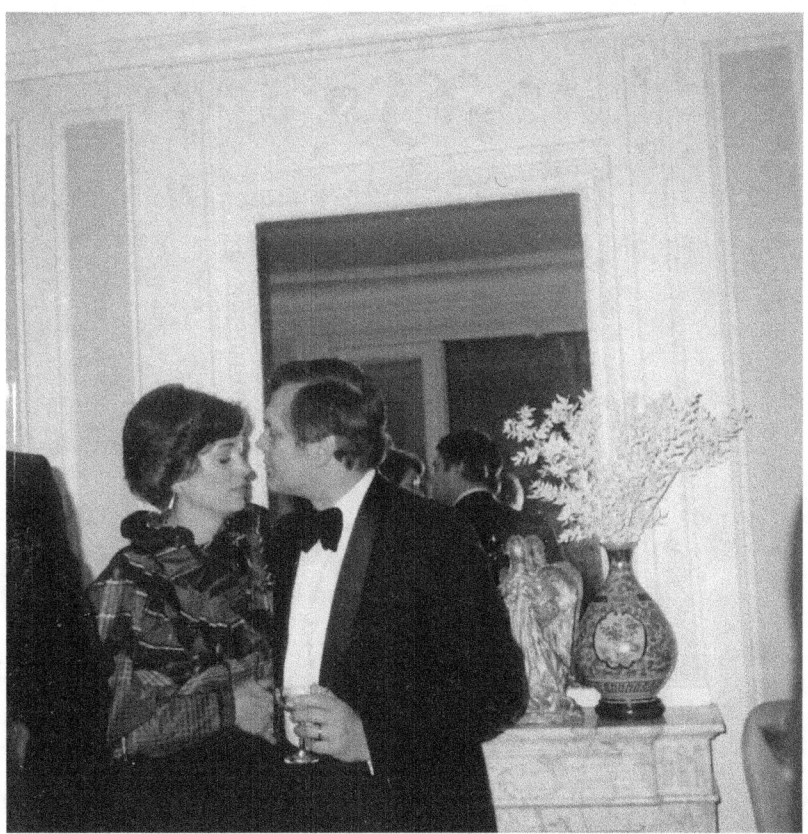

With Pat at New Year's Eve Party in Paris- 1981

CHAPTER 56
National Pride

One of the things that you learn early as an expatriate on an international assignment is to respect national pride. This applies both to the individuals that you may have working for you as employees, or those citizens with whom you may come in contact. Everyone is proud of their own country, and there are many stories of the "ugly American" berating some foreigner's comments or activities. So you definitely want to avoid that kind of behavior. Over the years I have had many examples of national pride, but two particularly stand out.

The first happened as I was returning to Hong Kong from Tokyo sometime early in my assignment, about ten years prior to the 1997 turnover of Hong Kong from British to Chinese rule. As was the custom for members of the regional staff, I was flying in business class, as opposed to the people that I knew on country level staffs who flew in coach. I remember that I was sitting in the front of the aircraft in the row ahead of an elderly, obviously British gentleman, who was travelling with a young boy that was probably his grandson. The flight into Hong Kong at that time was into Kai-Tak Airport, the airport famous for the aircraft passing dangerously by high-rise apartments on the Kowloon side of Hong Kong.

Kowloon was one of the most densely populated sections of the city, if not the world. After passing by the apartment complexes the plane then had to make a hard right turn into the center of the

Kowloon in order to reach the landing strip. (The airport has since been replaced by a much more modern facility on Lantau Island.) It was said that you could follow a television show in the windows of the high-rise apartments if you were seated on the right side of the aircraft.

Well, as we were nearing Hong Kong and had just made our approach to the Island, the gentleman looked out the window. The lights and majesty of the scene arriving in Hong Kong are nothing short of spectacular with the harbor and the high-rise buildings rising up the side of island. Suddenly he turned to his grandson and said, with a very pronounced British accent, "There it is my boy. Hong Kong! There is still something to be said for having a British passport." Touché for the Brits.

The second somewhat similar story happened in 1988 when I was making a flight from New Zealand to Sidney after doing some reviews of the banking territories in Auckland and Wellington. Again, I was in business class, sitting next to an Aussie that I had never met before. It turned out that he was one of the sponsors of one of the tall ships that had sailed into Sydney harbor during the 200th anniversary celebration earlier in the year. And it is true that the view of Sydney harbor from the air, with the opera house in full view, is quite spectacular. Well, as we passed over the harbor en-route to the Sydney airport, he turned to me and said, with a distinctly Australian accent, "You know, Mate. If you aren't living in Sydney, you're just camping out." Touché for the Aussies.

CHAPTER 57
I'll Ne'er Forget My College Days, part 3

Hong Kong International School was a good jumping off place for getting into a good college. It provided an excellent education for our children and also a excellent cultural experience for the students. There were students there from all over the world, and the interaction between the students was positive. They did not have cliques by grade but since most of the students were there for two to three years, associated more by the years that they were together, such as the classes of 1986-89. We had to make arrangements for Kelly to finish high school there, and it got a little tricky but we got it worked out.

Both of our children got into schools that suited them and for which they were well suited. Scott went to Colgate, in upstate New York, and Kelly to Georgetown, in Washington, DC. Scott was an economics major, and Colgate had an excellent Junior- year program in London. And Kelly was in the school of Languages and Linguistics, majoring in Mandarin.

The only thing that I would say about the differences in the schools was that Colgate was in a small, sleepy town, and once we paid for Scott's fraternity dues, there was not much else to do in the town on weekends but go to a fraternity beer party. Whereas in Georgetown, the sky was the limit. There were restaurants and discos all over town, and they were at Georgetown market prices. Many students there came from money. Perhaps the relationships that Kelly established in Georgetown made it worth it. And to be fair, she did get a part time job her senior year to make some spending money.

Scott joined Chase bank in NYC within several weeks of getting his Colgate degree in 1992, left Chase to get an MBA at Michigan in 1999 and now works at Bristol-Myers Squibb. He lives in Westfield, NJ with his wife, Cristina, and their three sons, Xavier, Rafael, and Felix.

After several unsuccessful starts, Kelly has landed an excellent job with ESPN in Hong Kong and regularly visits Beijing and Shanghai and speaks Mandarin as part of her responsibilities. So that has all worked out to her advantage. She is married to Ante Galic, another international manager from Toronto, and has a young son, Ante Wayne.

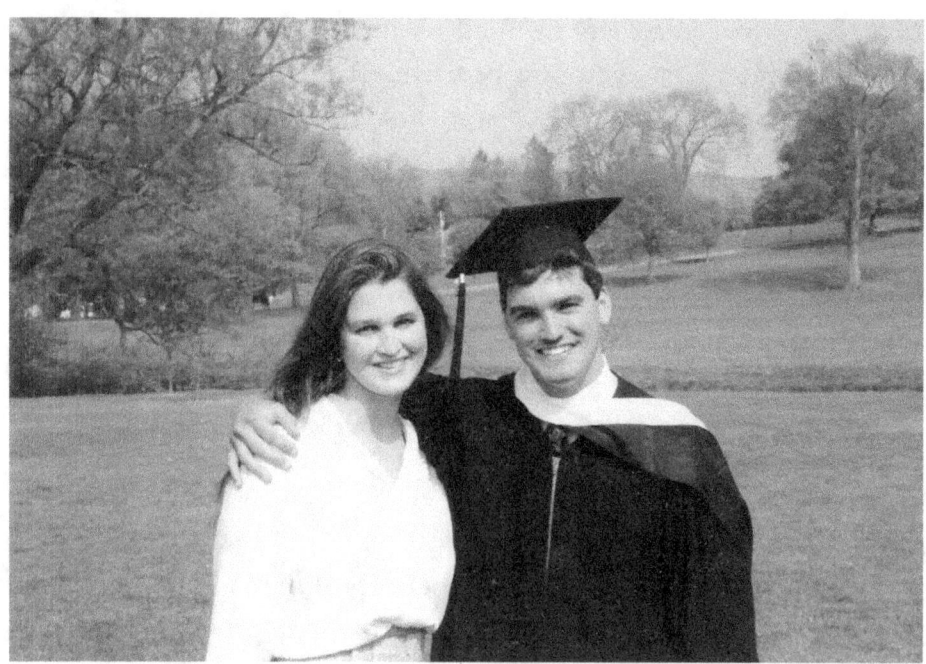

Scott and Kelly at Scott's Colgate University graduation-1992

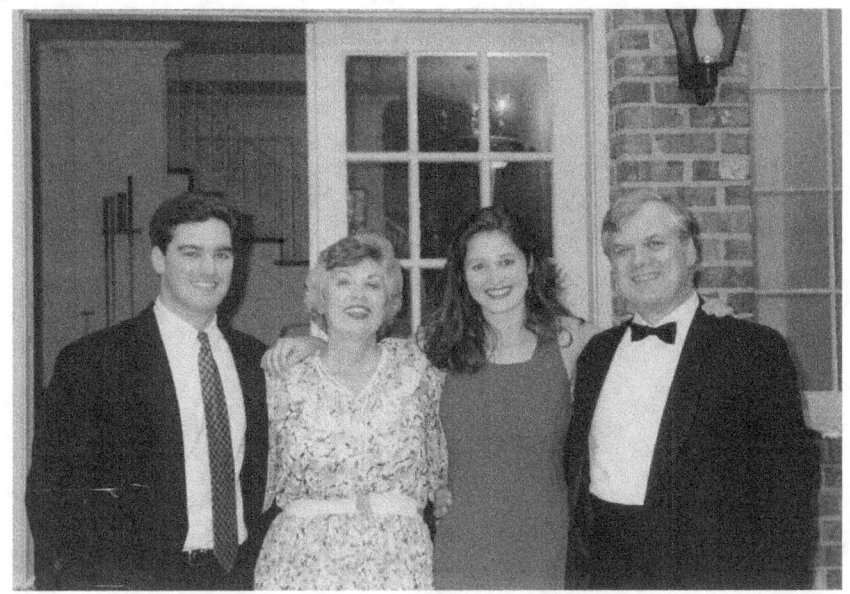

At Kelly's Georgetown graduation-1994

CHAPTER 58
The Finance Industry Reunion

After five years in Asia, John Bishop had moved back to Princeton, and we would see him and his wife, Dianne, socially on occasion. It was probably sometime in 1994 that we started the discussion on having a reunion of the Finance Industry Marketing team that John had managed in the 1970's. 1995 would mark the 20th anniversary of the re-launch of the 3600 Banking Terminals that was one of the high points of John's five years as Industry Director. John suggested that Clark Grimes, who had followed him as Industry Director when John had moved to Paris in 1979, would want to get involved in the discussions. Clark was living in Connecticut at the time. So we set up a dinner with our wives in nearby New Brunswick, New Jersey to start the discussion on the possibilities of a reunion.

Everyone was in favor of the possibilities, so it was just a matter of setting some ground rules and starting the work. There were not many of the Finance Industry IBMers living in the Princeton area any more since the industry had moved its headquarters to Charlotte, North Carolina in 1989. Others had moved to the White Plains, New York area. But it was felt that the reunion should be held in the Princeton area since that was where the Industry was located at the time John was the director.

John said that his executive secretary, Gretchen Yearick, still lived in the area and could be of help to us. It turned out that she was of excellent assistance, since she had copies of all of the old organization charts and also agreed to set up a bank account for the deposits. So we started to make a list of where people lived and find out if they were interested in attending. John agreed to write a letter to the people for whom we had addresses, which was about 50.

One thing led to another and soon I was creating a master database of names and addresses, and holding meetings on my screened-in porch. My wife and I checked out some hotels and selected the Scanticon Hotel which was located in Forrestal Center across College Road from the last location of the industry. Most of the people that we contacted were interested in coming if they could. And people who knew people helped us fill out our database of contacts, which soon grew to over a hundred names. It was a very positive response, and an indication of the respect that the Industry Staff had for John Bishop.

We scheduled the event for October 1995, set up a block of rooms at the hotel and started taking reservations. Over 75 industry alumni signed up and including spouses and guests the total number in attendance was about 130.

We got tickets for the Saturday afternoon Princeton University football game for those interested in attending, and set up a bar, buffet and disk jockey for the evening's festivities. Clark served as master of ceremonies and John gave an appropriate talk.

It was a great evening and a fun time was had by all. Everyone mentioned how they wished we had done it earlier and how they would like to do it again. As with events of that type, it was probably one of a kind.

I received a lot of kind comments regarding my role in the event and was very happy that I was able to help out. However, within a year, Bob Coates, one of the local staff, who had helped out with the planning, had passed away as did Herb Phillips, a Field Support Manager, who had worked for me and lived in Philadelphia. So it was timely that we were able to organize the event, schedule it and pull it off when we did.

CHAPTER 59
Coldwell Banker

In Hong Kong, my wife, Pat had worked with a company called Hong Kong Orientations that provided relocation orientation to new expat families moving into that area. She enjoyed that experience and so after returning to Princeton, she got involved with a relocation firm doing the same for people moving into the Greater Princeton Area. After doing that for a few years she decided to get her residential real estate license and started working for a local real estate firm. She was with them for a couple of years and started to have some success.

Then in the 1994, she did a number of deals with the local Coldwell Banker Princeton office and was encouraged to move to that firm at the end of the year. I had been working with an area consulting firm, and, early in 1995, Pat told me that she was getting busier with real estate and could use my help. She asked me if I would join her. So I proceeded to get my real estate license as well, and we started working together. We try to divide up the work so that she does more of the customer interaction and I do more of the computer and administrative work. And, if I must say so, we make an excellent team.

We have had some excellent years together in the business and it has only been recently when I have been somewhat slowed down by cancer that we have started to slow down in our production. But all in all, it has been a very good sixteen years for us. We have made a number of new friends through real estate, have had some excellent customers over the years, and now most of our business is done through referrals from current and prior customers.

CHAPTER 60
A Tribute to Lottie

In July of 1996 I received a call from the community nursing home in Bowling Green, Ohio. My mother, Lottie, was failing fast. She had moved into the home about seven years earlier when she had fallen and broken her hip. The home was located within view of her home on Ranch Court and she had often visited it in earlier years to teach crafts to the "old folks" when she was in her '80s. But now things were serious. I planned to drive out to meet up with my younger brother, Dan, who was planning to come from Dallas. I polled my children, Scott and Kelly, to see if either would want to join me in the ten hour drive across Pennsylvania to Bowling Green. Scott had more recently been in Bowling Green to see her, and was tied up at work. But Kelly had not been there for a while and decided to join up with me. My wife, Pat decided to stay behind until there was more definitive word on the situation.

So Kelly came down from New York and we started our drive around two o'clock in the afternoon, hoping to get to the nursing home to see Mom while she was still alive. Around midnight we pulled into Bowling Green and went right to the home after confirming that our reservation in the local Best Western was good. Mom was still alive, although we could tell that she was slowly leaving us. Her legs were starting to get cold. She did not recognize us and after a short visit, we decided to check into the hotel and get some sleep.

The next morning we went back to the nursing home. Mom was about the same. Dan had arrived and we left Kelly in the room with Mom while Dan and I discussed what arrangements we could make. We needed to talk to the United Methodist Church, where Mom had been a member for over 50 years, but which had a new minister that did not know her or the family. We needed to talk to the funeral home, which had handled Dad's arrangements and where one of the directors was in my high school class. We needed to think about writing an obituary for the newspapers. And we needed to alert our brother Allen, who was living and working in Hong Kong and about a day's flight away. So we made some phone calls and appointments, and left Kelly with Mom while we went to handle some arrangements, and actually picked out a casket at the funeral home. Later that day we checked back in with Kelly. No change in Lottie.

Mom remained stable for the next morning and her doctor said that her condition could remain the same for a number of days. Since Dan and I had done as much advance planning as we could, we decided to split and Kelly and I started the drive back to Princeton arriving late evening.

It was a day later when we got the call that we were dreading. Mom had passed away. She was 94 years old and had lived a very full life, which included sixteen grandchildren. She was a wonderful wife and mother, and even though she slowed down later in life, she was always singing as she rolled around in her wheelchair.

We held the service as planned and were surprised at the number of people that showed up that had read about it in the newspaper. She had a lot of friends in the community. Al and his wife, Molly, made it in from Hong Kong, although I am sure that they were at least somewhat jet-lagged for the service.

One thing that Mom had particularly requested was the playing of Dvorak's Largo (Going Home), which we included in the program. My brother, Jim, had a friend that lived in town and that evening we had a reception at his house for the family and guests. Ironically, the house was on North Prospect Street, next door to 445 where we had all grown up.

After the service, I realized that it was the end of an era. When both of your parents have passed on, you realize that you are, in fact, an orphan and are left to fend for yourself. I also realized that there would now be less incentive to visit Bowling Green, except, of course, to visit the cemetery where our parents are buried.

I found it difficult to sleep during the days we were getting ready for the service. Finally, after the service, I told my wife, Pat, that rather than going right back to Princeton; we should go to the Northern part of Michigan for a few days to rest up. She agreed and we drove north finally reaching Traverse City, on Grand Traverse Bay where we stayed for a couple of nights at the Bayshore Hotel.

We were right on the bay and with the door to the balcony of the room opened up we could feel the cool breezes of the night. That night I slept like a baby for the first time in days. It was a refreshing feeling and I realized that both Mom and Dad would not want me to languish at their departing, but to use their example to move forward in my life. And that is what I choose to do.

CHAPTER 61
Five Minutes of Fame

Many people dream about having their five minutes of fame in the media. Mine happened almost by accident. One day in the summer of 1999 I received a call from a producer of the NBC Early Show in New York about a segment they were making about retirees who may retire from their original employer but don't retire from the work-force. She had obtained my name from Steve McGrath, who was a colleague of mine when I worked at a local consulting firm and was now running an IT personnel search firm. Steve knew that I had taken an early retirement from IBM and was working with my wife in real estate. The producer wanted to know if I would be interested in being interviewed for the TV segment that they were developing. I said yes.

So it was a few weeks later that she and a cameraman showed up at our house in Princeton, New Jersey to film my part of the show. We found a good spot in the living room for the interview portion of the program and she explained the routine. She had a pre-determined list of questions that she would ask. I was sitting at an angle to the camera and would respond directly to the questions. There was no ad-hoc interaction.

The interview proceeded. She asked questions about retirement, and I explained that while I was officially retired from IBM that did not mean that I was not interested in working and continuing to make some money. I talked about the value of keeping good relations with the people that you had worked with in the past and networking with them. I thought that the interchange went fairly well, but it was fairly perfunctory.

After answering her questions, we went around the house to take some background shots of me working at my home computer and my wife and me walking with our dog, Toby, around the back yard. And after about an hour they were done and on their way back to NYC.

I didn't talk to the producer again. She had done her work and was moving on. But I did get a communication that the show would air on September 7, 1999 on MSNBC. My big claim to fame.

There was only one problem. It aired at 4:30 in the morning and I doubt if anyone I know saw it. So much for that. I have the tape if you are interested.

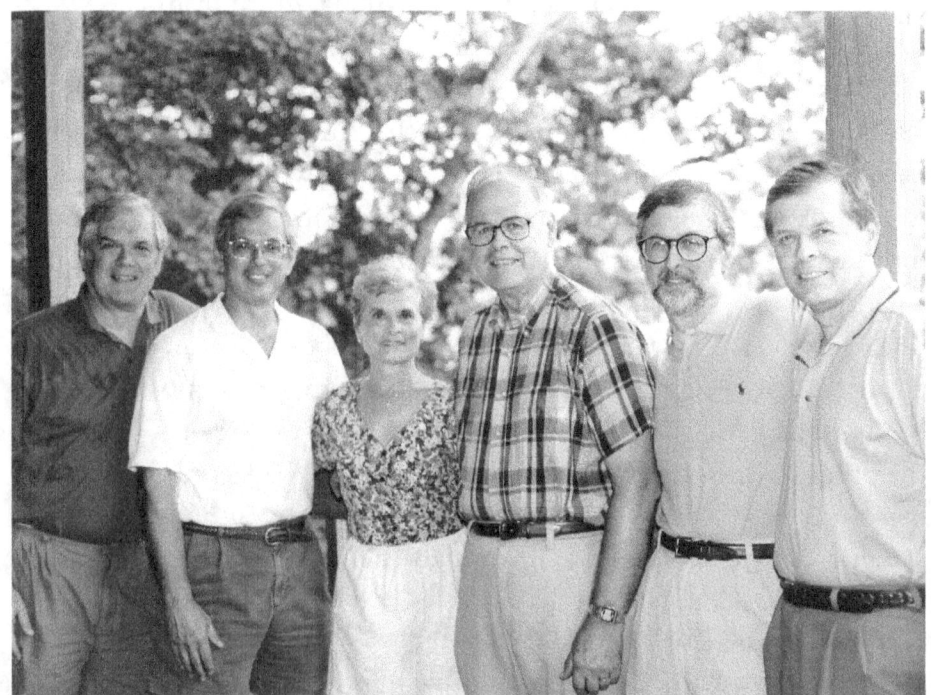

Wayne, Allen, Janet, Dean, Jim and Dan at family reunion- 1999

CHAPTER 62
Princeton United Methodist Church

After returning from Hong Kong, we had re-established our membership in the Princeton United Methodist Church. We had originally joined the church in the mid-'70s when our children had some friends who were members there, and I had been singing bass in the adult choir over the years.

In 1991, the then-chairperson of the Board of Trustees asked me if I would consider joining the board to complete the last year of a three-year term that was open because the person who had been voted in was moving. After discussing the details of the position, I agreed. It turned out that due to various circumstances, I would remain on the board for a total of ten years, the last three as chairperson. I then served an additional three years as the head of the capital funds campaign.

In 1993 we had started work on a campaign to replace the existing organ in the sanctuary. This resulted in the church organist and me making a visit to Red Bank, New Jersey, to examine a "gift" organ that was being donated to the church as part of an estate. It was in pieces in the donor's basement. The donor was building it himself and little of it was put together, especially the console. After some due diligence by people more knowledgeable than me on church organs, our church decided to accept the gift, hired a professional to assemble it, and it is now an essential part of our sanctuary.

Then in 1996, we added an experienced architect to our board and started discussions on the renovation of our existing one-story education building. I won't get into all of the details, but we selected an architectural firm to develop plans and proceeded to select a contractor to demolish the interior of the then-existing structure and build a new two-story education facility.

From 1997 to 2000 I was the chair of the Board of Trustees and one of the church point people for the project, along with a team of three other people; our minister, Rev. James Harris, the architect, Tim Winstead, and George Lee, a member of the board. Our team was active about six years. Over those six years we optimistically started the project, saw work progress, then had to fire the first contractor, hired another contractor, and went to arbitration over our increased costs. We won the arbitration suit, only to lose our battle for financial relief from the sub-contractors. It was a trying time. But things recovered in 2003 when the settlement of an estate brought us the money needed to pay off all of the construction debt. And the building has been a well-used asset for the church ever since.

I cannot be more proud of the work that all of the church teams did to bring about the completion of the education building project. And along with the scholarship fund for my parents, it is one of the significant achievements of my life. I believe that my planning skills played a major part in the success of these two projects.

CHAPTER 63
Carnegie Hall

How do you get to Carnegie Hall? In the joke, the response is "Practice, my boy, practice." In my case it was due to the Voices Chorale, an audition-based, mixed chorus in the Princeton, New Jersey- Bucks County, Pennsylvania area that I have belonged to since it started in the early 1990's. I have made three singing trips to Europe with them: to Bavaria, Germany in 1999, to Germany and Austria in 2003 and to Germany and Northern Italy and Venice in 2007. And I have sung with them in Carnegie Hall not once, not twice, but three times.

There is an organization in New York City called Mid-American Productions that specializes in promoting trips to the city for choruses from around the US and other countries. Mid-American will coordinate tours of the city, and arrange for the rehearsals and a concert in Carnegie Hall of a major chorale work. About five or six choruses will be combined to perform the work. Often the producer of the event is concerned about the professionalism of the choruses that are involved. And that is where the Voices Chorale comes in.

Our director, Lyn Ransom, knows the producer of these events and on occasion arranges for our chorale to learn the works, if we do not know them already, and, for those members that are interested, to go to NYC for the rehearsals and then perform the work with the visiting choruses in Carnegie Hall.

So I have done that three times; first to sing the Durufle Requiem in 2001; then to sing Part 3 of the Messiah (which is not frequently done) in 2002; and, finally, to sing a new work by Bob Chilcott, a British composer in 2007.

And a nice extra thing about it was that my daughter, Kelly, had sung the Durufle Requiem at Georgetown, so I arranged with Lyn for her to sing with us. So father and daughter had the opportunity to sing together at Carnegie Hall in the April, 2001 concert. What a treat.

When you walk out onto that stage, you have to feel a bit of awe when you think of all of the famous composers, conductors and artists that have walked there before you. It is an amazing experience and one in which you hope you do justice to the work that you are performing. I believe that we did.

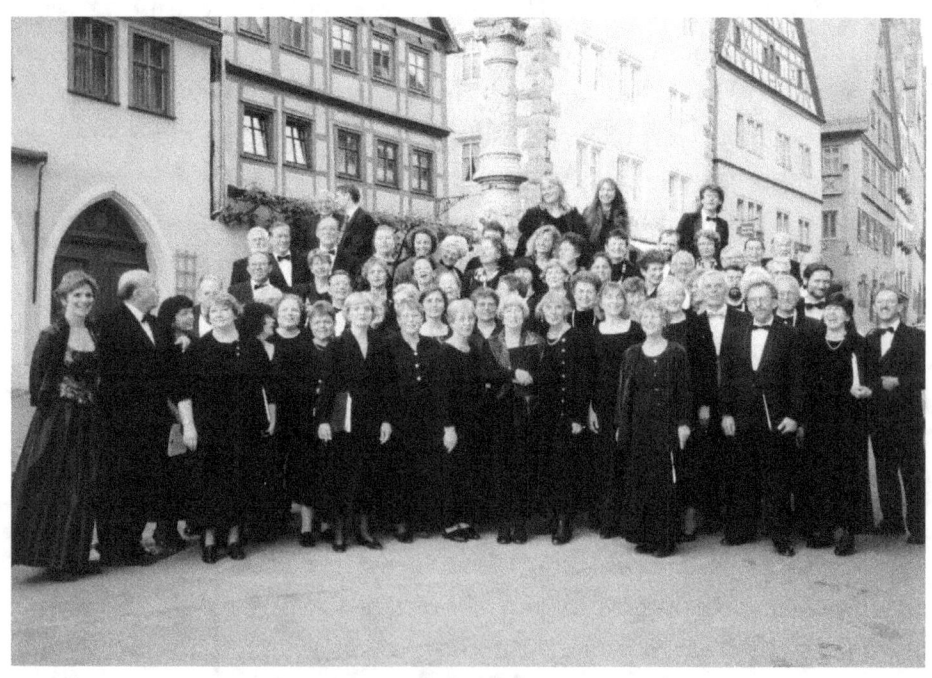

Voices Chorale in Rothenburg, Germany- 1999

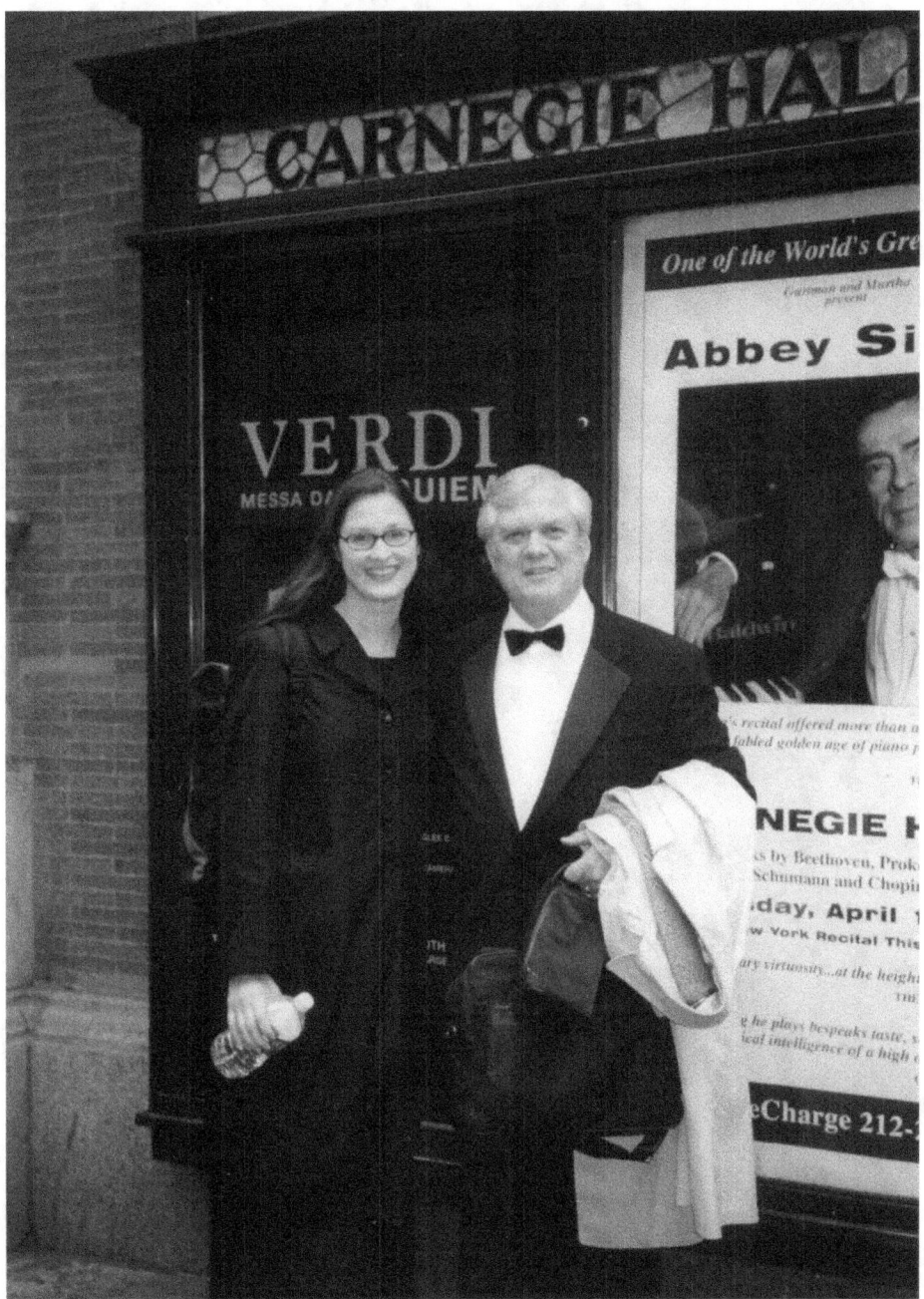

With Kelly after singing together in Carnegie Hall- April 2001

CHAPTER 64
Five Dogs and a Cat

Pat grew up in a family that had dogs. My family did not have any pets in our home until after I had graduated from high school when my brothers got a couple of hamsters. So after Pat and I were married and had settled in our new home in Pittsburgh, one of the first things she wanted to do was to get a dog. That was the first of five dogs and one cat that we would eventually own.

I decided that if we were going to get a dog it should be a pure bred. Pat decided on a German Schnauzer. We visited a local breeder and she was proud that the dog we were looking at was the offspring of a Western Pennsylvania champion. We bought the dog and named him the Baron von Fritzen. We thought that a fancy German dog should have a fancy German name. His nickname was Fritts.

Fritts was also frisky. There was a female Schnauzer that lived down the hill from us in the North Hills of Pittsburgh. There were times when Fritts would jump right through the screen door in our family room, run down the hill to the house where the female lived, and on occasion, if the screen door there was closed, jump through the door there, chase the dog around the dining room table and chase her out into the back yard where he would perform whatever came naturally.

We knew all this because we would get a call from the owner of the female, suggesting that we get together to pray over the dogs. I did not care to get together to pray, but I had checked out the cost of getting screen doors repaired and offered to pay her for the cost of getting it done.

Our Schnauzer's updated nickname was Fritts the Skitts. When Scott was a baby, he slept well at night. But our daughter Kelly had colic. They say when your child has colic they outgrow it in three months. If they don't, then they will outgrow it in six months. Kelly was one of the six months type. She cried all night, most nights. So we went through about six months when one of us was up all night walking with the baby. She would then sleep a bit during the day, but if anyone came to the door and rang the bell, Fritts the Skitts would bark like crazy and wake Kelly up.

It got to the point where we decided we had to get rid of either the dog or the baby for the sake of our sanity. We chose to get rid of the dog. We put an ad in the local paper and got a taker. We were willing to give the dog away for nothing, although we had paid a pretty good price for it. I delivered the dog to the recipient and did receive a handful of dollars in return. I have to admit that I shed a little tear when I drove away from the transfer.

We got our one cat, Angel as a kitten when Kelly was three years old, and it lived for fourteen years. We got her at Christmas and to keep it a secret, we asked a neighbor to keep the cat at her house until Christmas day. When the neighbor's mother, who was visiting for Christmas, saw the cat, she asked her daughter how it happened that she had a cat. Her daughter replied, "Oh it's the Cooke's cat." And the mother replied. "Well I am so glad that you have finally gotten some household help."

There are a lot of stories about Angel, but probably the best one is when we were getting ready to move to Holland. Pat talked to the local kennel people about whether she needed shots prior to the move. The people said no. Time passed and finally we were about a month before we were to fly out. I asked Pat to check again. They said no shots required. Then two weeks later, I asked Pat to ask them about taking a cat into the Netherlands. They said "Yes" shots are required to take a cat into the Netherlands, but not Holland. Someone here needs a geography lesson. We were too late to make the required date for the shots, but got them anyway and decided we would try to gut out any problems with quarantine.

When we arrived in Schiphol Airport for our entry into The Netherlands, we had two adults, two children, eight suitcases, three carry-on bags and one cat case (with Angel inside) loaded onto several baggage carts. We rolled up to the customs officials and they waved us through. Welcome to the Netherlands. Er, I mean Holland. And she prevailed for five adventurous years in Europe.

Angel did not go with us to Hong Kong because we were told that she would have had to go into quarantine for six months, and many pets did not survive. So we "boarded" her with my brother, Jim, in Montclair, New Jersey for the three years and picked her up on our return. She survived until 1990.

We had a couple of other dogs before going to Hong Kong, but after we returned from Hong Kong, we were without a dog for a while. Then Pat and a friend both decided that they wanted to get a collie. Pat found a collie breeder in central Jersey and we visited her and picked out a male from several litters that she had. We bought this dog as a puppy and named him Toby-wan Kenobi, Toby for short. He became an excellent pet and we had him for twelve years.

After Toby, Pat did not wait too long to have him replaced. The breeder we had bought Toby from was no longer in business, and after one unsuccessful venture, in 2002 we found another collie breeder on the road down to Atlantic City. She also had several litters of collies, and we picked a dog from the bunch and named him Luke. We still have Luke and he has also been an excellent dog. It is interesting that two collies, Toby and Luke, could look so much alike and yet have such different attributes. But both were fine dogs.

I have to admit that after living over forty years with pets, I have a much better appreciation for them and particularly enjoy having Luke around. He has developed into a very compatible dog.

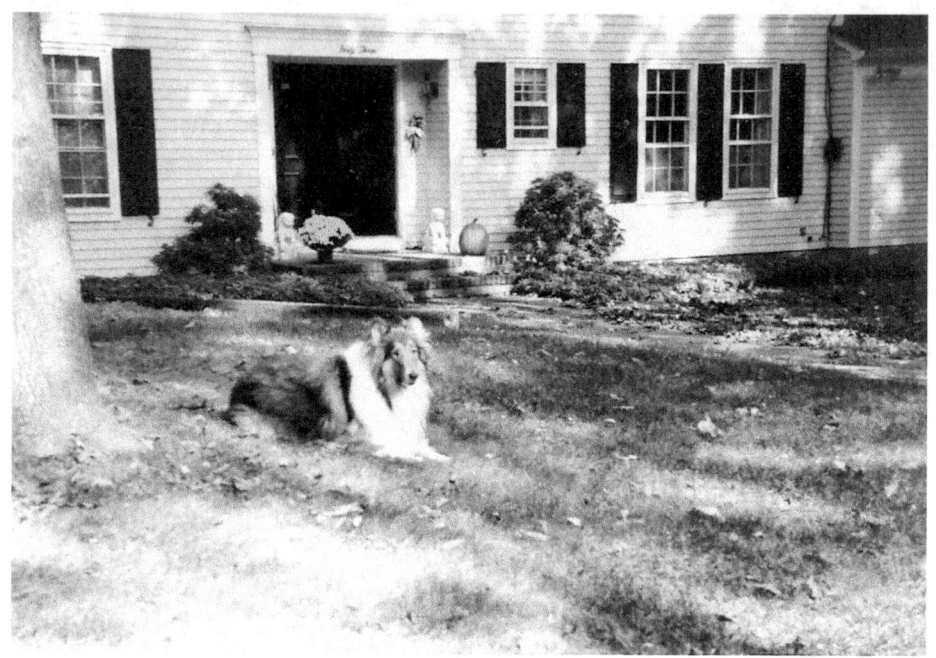

Toby at 43 Beech Hill Circle

CHAPTER 65
The Year 2008

The year 2008 was a special year for the Wayne Cooke family for a number of reasons

First, in April, Pat and I celebrated our 40th wedding anniversary by cashing in some Marriott award points and staying for a week in Paris. We were at the Renaissance Hotel near Place Vendome in the central part of city. It was a great location within walking distance of the Louvre and a wonderful way to revisit some of our favorite haunts and restaurants.

Next, in June my wife, Pat, and I continued the celebration with a party on our deck with a number of our family and friends in attendance. We had it catered by a local firm and hired a piano player who was tinkling on the ivories in the corner of the deck on her portable keyboard. Of course there was a large cake. And then our children, Scott and Kelly, surprised us with a blown-up poster of us walking down the aisle of the Shrine of the Little Flower in Royal Oak, Michigan in June 1968. They also used the same photo for special champagne glasses that they had made up. Kelly had flown in from Hong Kong just for the occasion. It was one of the best parties we have ever enjoyed.

And it was just a few weeks later that my wife surprised me with a birthday party on my 75th birthday. She had me going over to a neighbor's house for some trumped up chore while she was getting ready and the guests were arriving. I try to stay alert to those types of things, but I have to admit that I was totally caught off guard by her varkiness in the matter and again, it was a wonderful time.

We were also blessed that year that in spite of the economic downturn in the US, both of our children had good jobs, Scott with Bristol-Myers Squibb in New Jersey and Kelly with ESPN in Hong Kong.

And Xavier, our grandson in Westfield, NJ was on track to successfully complete the second year of his three year treatment schedule for childhood leukemia.

Then our daughter, Kelly, invited us to spend that Thanksgiving with her in Hong Kong. The visit included a side trip to the Renaissance Resort Hotel in Koi Samui, a small island off of the east coast of Thailand. So it was a wonderful trip.

And by the end of the year, I had completed five years as a cancer survivor.

So as Frank Sinatra would say. "It was a very good year."

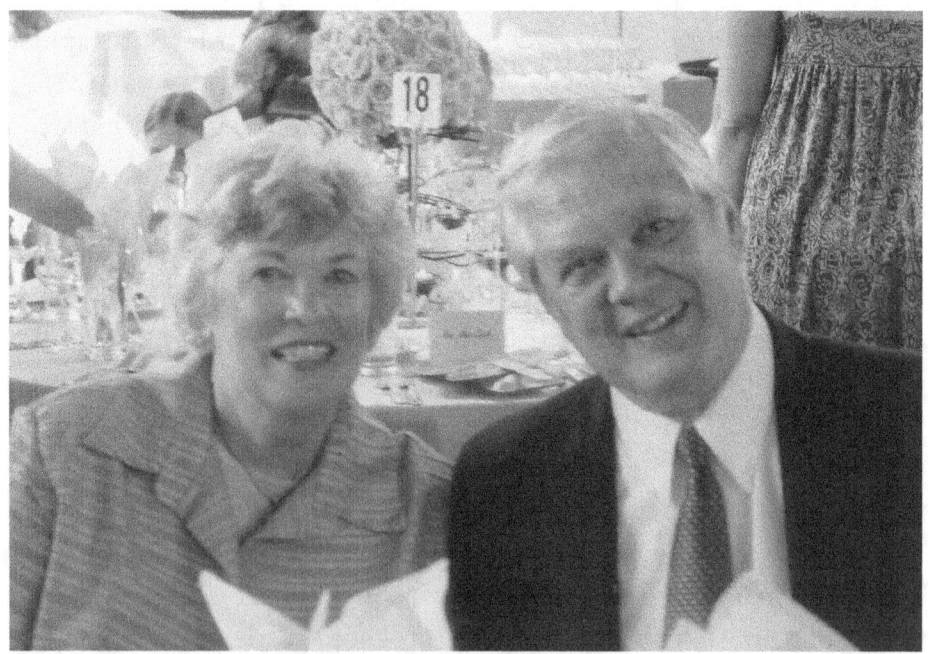

With Pat at wedding in Dallas

CHAPTER 66
Music, The International Language

It is the summer of 2003 and I am singing a concert with Voices Chorale and the Chorus of the St. Sebald Roman Catholic Church of Erlangen, Germany in the church sanctuary. A soprano member of the St. Sebald group had moved to the Princeton area with her husband in the late 1990's, and joined the Voices Chorale. When she later moved back to Germany she helped arrange for our two choirs to sing together. We did three tours of Germany and other countries with their chorus and their chorus did one tour to the states with us.

This was our second experience of singing together in Germany; the first was in 1999 and there was to be a later one in 2007. On this trip we had performed together in Nuremburg and other surrounding locations and we were performing this concert for the church congregation before heading off for Salzburg, Austria. The music was primarily from German composers of the area and so was primarily in German with a bit of Latin thrown in. We rehearsed the music together but normally sat in our own groups for rehearsal. At the concert, however, the choruses were intermixed and I found myself standing in the back row beside a German bass singer whom I had not met before. The concert went off without a hitch and I enjoyed standing next to the German gentleman, whose pronunciation of the language helped keep me on track. At the end of the concert, I turned to him and told him in English how much I had enjoyed singing next to him.

I quickly realized that he did not understand a word that I was saying. We had been standing together and singing together for the better part of an hour, and yet if we tried to talk to each other it would have been extremely difficult. On the other hand we were able to sing the music together without any difficulty at all and enjoyed each other's presence while doing do. It was a demonstration of the power of music to transcend our difficulties in communicating by language. I thought that if more people could do this, what a wonderful world it would be.

Moving ahead to May 2011, Pat and I are in Xi'an, China to see the terra-cotta warriors of the Qin Dynasty. We had been visiting our daughter, Kelly and her newborn son in Hong Kong and had planned this side trip that we had always wanted to take but were not able to do so while we lived in Asia.

While planning the trip, I had mentioned it to Jie Hayes, a soprano member of the Methodist Church choir where I sing. She amazed me by stating that she had grown up in Xi'an and that her parents were still living there. Her father was the conductor of a Chinese chorus and her mother was an instrumentalist on the Pipa, a Chinese stringed instrument. Jie was excited about our going to her hometown and contacted her parents who invited us to have dinner with them while we were there. The only problem was that they did not speak any English. But Jie said that her sister, who lived in Xi'an, did and could help translate.

So on a Friday evening in Xi'an, Pat and I are waiting in the lobby of the Shangri-La Hotel to meet with Jie's parents. They arrive on schedule, are very cordial and take us to a restaurant where they have arranged for a private room for us to have dinner with the daughter and another couple that fortunately spoke excellent English. We had a wonderful time. During the meal I talked to the father through his daughter about his music, and at the end of the meal it becomes apparent that he is conducting a rehearsal for his chorus on Saturday afternoon. We have no plans for that time and I ask him if I could attend the rehearsal. He is delighted and says that he would be pleased to have me attend and will arrange for me to be picked up at the hotel

Saturday comes and he arrives at the hotel with one of the basses of his chorus, who speaks pretty good English. Well, when we arrive at the rehearsal hall, he has me placed on the stage before his mixed chorus of about 70 members. They rehearse several numbers in Chinese, then Latin, German and English. They were also doing a number by Felix Mendelssohn, the German composer. I ask for a copy of the music and sing along with them. Then Jie's father asks me to sing a solo. I gracefully decline but agree to address the chorus in English. So I make some comments about how the music that they sing is very similar to what we might sing in the states and so forth, which are translated in Chinese to the crowd.

And as I am leaving to be driven back to the hotel, they applaud and then start singing another song that I happen to know. I poke my head back into the hall and join in the singing. They applaud again. Finally I am able to leave. What an experience. I am able to join in singing with an all-Chinese chorus knowing barely a word of Chinese. And they are thrilled. And when we arrive back home in Princeton, Jie tells me that she has heard from her parents about how delighted they were to meet with us. Another example of how music transcends language.

And music transcends generations as well. If you have ever sung Handel's" Messiah" in a community chorus with teenagers intermixed with the grandparents, you know that they all get joy out of singing good music together.

Where there is good music, there is joy; whatever country you are from and whatever your age. I am now 78 years old and still enjoy singing. I tell my daughter, Kelly, who is about half my age and has a very good voice, that if she keeps up her singing skill, she can find enjoyment in it for the rest of her life.

And so can you. If you have any musical skill, use it.

CHAPTER 67
Using Your Skills

My father, Gilbert, was a big proponent of using the skills and attributes that you have been given in life. He would say that everyone has been given some skills and no two people have been given the same skills, but the important thing is to figure out what yours are and use them over the course of your life. And please, don't waste them.

A couple of paragraphs from my first book *On the Far Side of the Curve: a Stage IV Colon Cancer Survivors Journey* helped to expand on this thought.

"He (Gilbert) was a firm believer in the value of education as well as the need to use the skills that you have been given. He used to tell the story of two students: Both got Bs on an exam, but they were not the same. One student was a C-level student so his B grade was an excellent performance for him. The other student was an A level student so his B grade was a wasted performance. The message of the parable: use your skills- don't waste them.

He strongly imparted those values to his six children. He did not have to say much. Just a few words and the look on his face were all it took to show either his pleasure or displeasure with your performance.

I think that my siblings and I spent a good part of our early lives seeking acceptance from our father. And maybe that search for acceptance helped establish a positive attitude in each of us."

I have been giving some thought to the skills that I have been given in life. I believe that one has core skills that you are born with and just need to nurture, and then there are the acquired skills that you develop over your life. I have come up with a list of nine skills that I believe that I have; two core and seven acquired skills.

Here are the nine skills:

Two Core skills.

Music: I consider my first core skill to be the love of music and singing. I have made several references in these memoirs about my love of music. I have enjoyed music as long as I can remember and believe that I have been especially good at singing from a very early age. Over the course of my life I have sung in junior high and high school choruses, church choirs, university choruses and men's glee clubs, musical comedies, barbershop choruses and quartets, folk song groups, and classical music choruses. At one time I was fairly decent in playing the ukulele and the banjo. I have been fortunate enough to sing in a number of musical venues including three times in Carnegie Hall. And, of course, I enjoy listening to music from the early days of vinyl recordings on 78, 45, or 33 1/3 rpm to the CDs of today. Music is a love that I will enjoy for the rest of my life.

Mathematics: My second core skill is mathematics. Many people would say that music and mathematics are inter-related since music theory is based on mathematical relationships and many people who are good in the one skill are also good in the other. I probably started to stand out in mathematics in grade school, but in high school I would have to say that I excelled. As I remember, I was always among the top scorers in the class. And when I started at the University of Missouri, I listed my major as Mathematics. I did quite well my first year, but in my sophomore year I had a lapse during my advanced calculus final and my grade dropped from an A to a B, the only B that I received in a math course during my four years of college. I decided then that maybe mathematics was not my best choice of majors and switched to business administration at Michigan.

I had turned my love of math over the years into a pretty good sense for bridge playing and I used that attribute during my time at boy scout camp, at college and during many social gatherings while on overseas assignments. I have also enjoyed solving puzzles such as Sudoku. And I think a math background was a definite asset in my thirty years at IBM

Seven Acquired skills

Swimming: I learned to swim at an early age and, during junior high, took swimming and life saving lesions at the Bowling Green State University pool. After my short spell at trying competitive racing while in the NROTC, I have reverted to social swimming and have enjoyed a backyard pool with my family for over twenty-five years.

Love of Travel: As I mentioned earlier in this story, I had done little travel out of Northwestern Ohio until after high school. It was during NROTC cruises that I first experienced international travel and that continued during my Naval service. Since those early days, I have been fortunate to live in three countries, The Netherlands, France, and Hong Kong and have gone overseas on three singing tours. In spite of my cancer, I have been able to make international trips since 2007.

Theatrical Ability: I did a bit of theatrical work in high school, but it was not until I went to Jackson, Michigan in 1960 and joined the Clark Lake Players that I really blossomed. Gaining experience there helped me to get roles with the Jackson Gilbert & Sullivan Society, The Birmingham Village Players in Birmingham, Michigan, the North Star Players in Pittsburgh, and the McCarter Theater in Princeton, New Jersey. My wife, Patricia, who was a speech and drama major in college, and I were fortunate enough to perform together in Birmingham, Michigan and Pittsburgh.

Planning/Organizing: You get a start on these skills in the Navy, but you can't spent 30 years at IBM without developing some planning and organizational skills. I used those skills when I was helping to initiate the Gilbert and Lottie Cooke Memorial Scholarship Fund at Bowling Green State University and when I was active in leadership positions at the Princeton United Methodist Church. They also helped when I was assisting my wife during my 15 years in residential real estate.

Positive attitude/ Determination: I believe that I have had a positive attitude about my life since high school and just continued in that development while in the Navy and in IBM. I believe that having a positive mental attitude is paramount in dealing with a disease such as cancer.

Parenting: The only training that you can get for this skill is "on the job training." And the only way you can measure this skill is looking back on it in hindsight. Well, my wife, Patricia, and I have raised two children, Scott and Kelly. As we look back on how their lives evolved, I believe that we could look at ourselves and say "Well done." Scott is now approaching forty-two and Kelly just turned thirty-nine. They both have good jobs, good marriages and healthy children. What more could you ask for?

Varking: I think that you have heard enough about my inquisitiveness and my varking abilities. Enough said.

I have made reference to these skills as we have progressed through the chapters of this book so you should have some idea about how they have played out in my life. If you are a close friend or relative of mine, you might debate whether I actually have these skills. What I say to that is that you are entitled to your own opinion. Perhaps you can think about your own skills and how you have used them as well. Please don't waste them.

CHAPTER 68
The Red Sport Coat

Pete Brower was always well dressed when he came to church. He was a member of the Princeton United Methodist Church that I had known since I was on the board of trustees with his wife, Mary Jo, in the early 90's. And he and I were on a church committee together in 1993 when we needed to select a new organ for the sanctuary.

About ten years later, I started to notice when he came to church on some special occasions wearing a beautiful red sport coat. I used to remark to him how handsome he looked. He always dressed well but with the red sport coat it was something special and you could always pick him out in his regular seat in the back of the sanctuary.

I had mentioned in my first book how I always am planning for the future and that has helped me take my mind off the daily aspects of living with cancer. It was in the fall of 2007 that I remarked to my wife, Pat, that if I survived cancer for another year, I wanted to treat myself by buying a red sport coat.

Well I did survive for another year and bought the coat at the end of 2008. I wear it now at Christmas, for Valentine's Day, and for other special occasions and feel very sporty doing so. If people come up to me to remark about my peacock-like appearance, I comment on how the coat is a remembrance to me of my cancer survivorship which I feel is a positive thing. I would hope that my wearing the coat would have the same influence on them as Pete wearing his coat did on me.

And now I have just started to plan for a special birthday celebration in July 2013 so I will need to survive at least until that date. It is a red sport coat type event, but it will probably be too warm to wear it. Stay tuned.

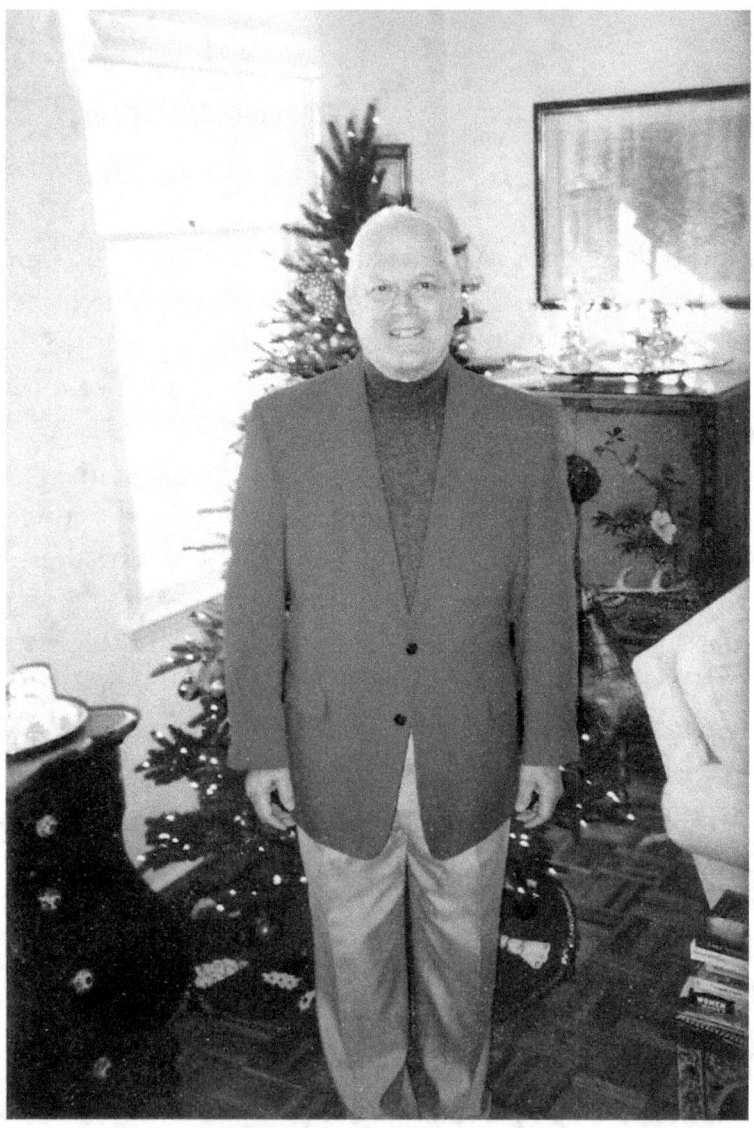

The Red Sport Coat

CHAPTER 69
A Fresh Look At Cancer

In November 2011, I will have completed eight years as a Stage IV Colon Cancer survivor. It is almost impossible to believe but true. My first book *On the Far Side of the Curve: A Stage IV Colon Cancer Survivors Journey*, published in December 2009, covered the first six years of that survivorship.

I have had more chemo than I ever thought imaginable, over 130 different sessions of five different regimes. And my most recent cocktails were not even available when I first started chemo in February 2004. So progress is being made in cancer treatments. The longer that you can survive, the more treatments become available. And since I am in an incurable status, I will probably be on some kind of chemo for the rest of my life.

For most of this year my treatments were every other week with manageable side effects. I would have scans about every three months and live from scan to scan; hopeful that the spots have shrunk. My scans in May 2011 were stable. But my scans in October showed that some spots are growing, so I have now started on a clinical trial at the Cancer Institute of New Jersey. It is a new drug that is now yet on the market. I will have my next scans in January to see how I am doing.

When I think back on my life, and all that I have been fortunate enough to do, I realize that today I am probably living on borrowed time and that the cancer could get worse at any scan. I feel, however, that I have made and will continue to make good use of my skills. Hopefully, my father, Gilbert, would not think that I have wasted them.

I have no complaints about my current situation with cancer and have no fears about what the future holds. I will deal with it as it comes, a day at a time following the advice of my oncologist, Dr. Peter Yi.

I wrote in my first book that I found inspiration from Isaiah Chapter 40 Verse 31 that said "But they that wait upon the Lord will renew their strength: they shall mount up with wings as eagles: they shall run, and not be weary: they shall walk, and not faint." I recited that passage to myself as I was being rolled into surgery or undergoing a particularly arduous test.

What I believe now is that I could not have made it this far as a Stage IV survivor without a higher being looking after me. Doctors tell me that my survival is remarkable, that I am a "unique individual," and a "Miracle Man." So I have started to take a view of my survival that looks to the 23rd Psalm verse 4. "Yea though I walk through the valley of the shadow of death, I will fear no evil: for thou art with me: thy rod and thy staff they comfort me." I truly believe that the power of the Holy Spirit is in me. Someone upstairs wants me to survive and to use my example and learning experience for the good of others.

Therefore, what I am finding is that my being a cancer survivor for so long is resonating in a positive way with a number of people. Over the past three years or so I have made contact with well over a dozen people who are dealing with or have had various cancers. For them, I am an example of a successful outcome and they appreciate my communications.

Although their cancers may not be the same that I have, the fact that I have been successful so far has provided hope and inspiration to them, their caregivers and their families. And I am beginning to think that this is a new skill that I can develop and a new role that I can play in my life; to be an example for others by supporting them in their individual fights against cancer. And in doing so to help pay back for all of the support that I have had in my own personal fight against cancer. It would be my tenth skill and is something that I feel would be worthwhile for me to do. And hopefully, I could do it well.

Not all of these cancer patients have made it. But I hope that my involvement with them and their caregivers has made their journeys easier. And it has made me more resolute as well to succeed in my journey, along with my help from above.

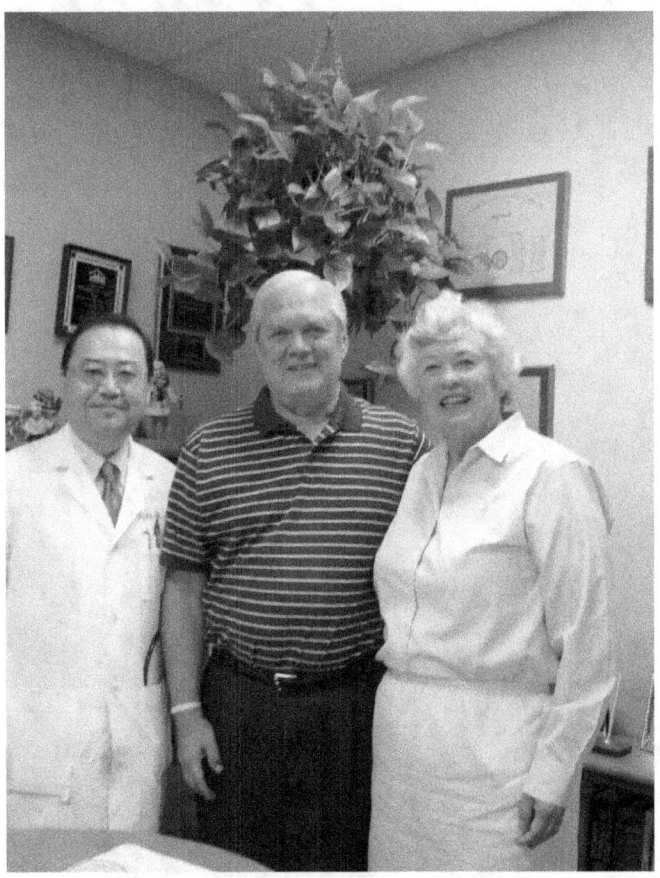

With Pat and Dr. Yi-August 2009

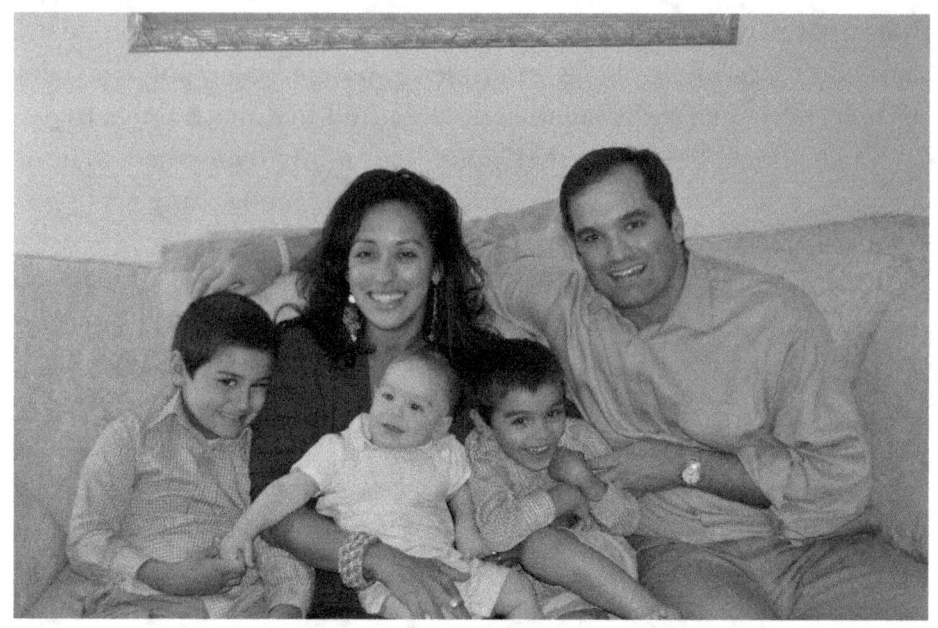

Scott's family

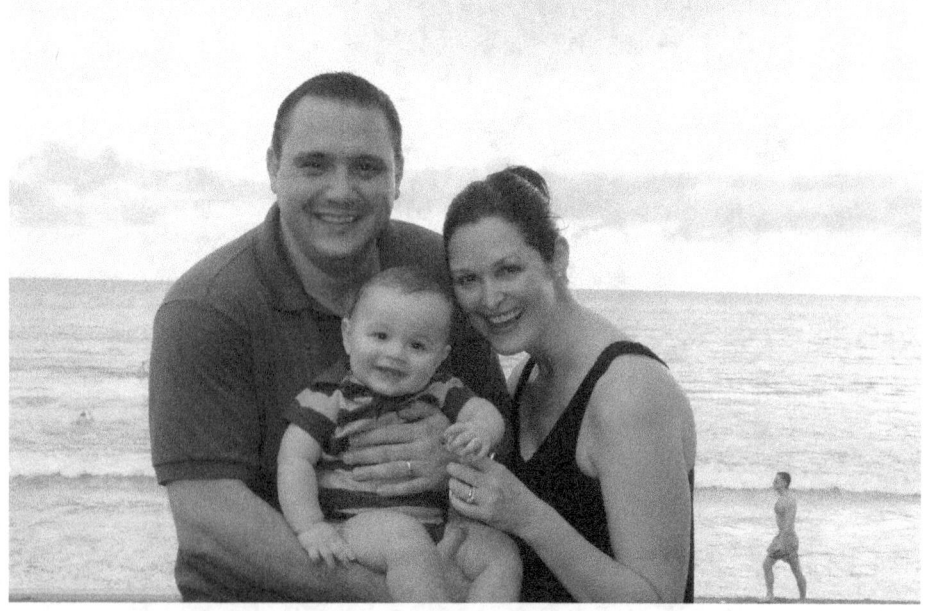

Kelly's family

CHAPTER 70
Lessons Learned

I originally planned to end this book with the previous chapter. But on preparing for a radio interview about my previous book *On The Far Side Of The Curve,* I realized that Chapter 17 of that book entitled "Lessons Learned" might be an appropriate ending for this book as well. There I incorporated fourteen lessons based on my cancer experience that I thought might be helpful for other cancer survivors or for others dealing with serious illnesses. So I have decided to use those lessons, in some cases modified to remove the specific cancer references, as the basis for this chapter. I have also added two additional lessons that I have thought of since I wrote the first book. I believe that these lessons are valid, not only for dealing with cancer, but for living life as well.

"LESSON 1: THE CAREGIVER

It is important to have a caregiver to support you when you are dealing with cancer or any other serious disease, and my wife, Pat, has done an exceptional job in that capacity. She has gone with me for most of my consultations with my oncologist, my surgeons, and specialists. Having two sets of ears hearing the advice makes it more likely that you will agree on the process going forward. She was also invaluable in helping me recover from three surgeries, helping button and unbutton my shirts when I was dealing with the neuropathy that I developed from my first chemo regime, and letting me nap when I've been fatigued from chemotherapy.

I hope that you, the reader, do not have to go through a disease or illness that necessitates having a caregiver, but if you do, I hope that yours is as good as my wife has been to me.

LESSON 2: THE MEDICAL TEAM

I believe that I have had the best medical team that you could find and that without the knowledge and dedication of my doctors and specialists, I would not be here today. You may not be in need of a medical team in your life today, but I would submit anyone going through life today is in need of some specialists to assist them. They may need doctors, lawyers, tax experts, brokers, financial planners, ministers or any number of specialist skills. So it is important for anyone to identify the skills that they may need to assist them in life and have those skills lined up in advance.

We, for example, have made sure that my wife, Pat, is comfortable not only with my doctors, but also with our financial planners, and with our will and estate attorney. So at the present time, we have not only the medical team to deal with but also various other experts. As long as Pat is happy and content with the team, I am as well.

You may be in need of other types of specialist skills than my wife and I are, but I would encourage you to discuss the needs openly and line up the support that you need in advance of an emergency situation. Build the best team that you can.

"LESSON 3: HAVING A PLAN

It's been said that when you don't know where you are going, any road will take you there. When you have a plan, you have some purpose in your life. We have found that when we knew what was on the docket for my treatment schedule for the next month or two, it made living day by day much easier and just a step in the direction of the plan. And each good day that you have continues to build up your memories of the past.

I have been keeping annual plans ever since we have been married, for 43 years now, long before I developed cancer. Having cancer for the past eight years has made some modifications for those plans, but has not changed the concept in any way. As they used to say at IBM, "Plan your work, and work your plan."

LESSON 4: KEEP THE FAITH BABY

I have found that keeping the church involved in all aspects of my journey has been very beneficial to me. From the church prayer chain that has prayed for the success of my surgeries and treatments to the personal visitations from our senior pastor to the joy I have found in singing in the choir, to the Thursday small group bible study, to the daily prayers that my wife and I share, we have found strength in keeping our faith.

Our minister, Dr. Greg Young, frequently prayed with me for the healing touch of the Lord and visited us both at home and in the hospitals in Princeton and NYC. My faith started as far back as my early days in Bowling Green, Ohio when my mother would dress up all of her children in their Sunday best and we would walk the four blocks to the Methodist Church and take up a row of eight: mom and dad, and the six children. This was normally followed by a typical Sunday dinner, with, perhaps, one or two of my father's students in attendance.

One bible verse which I have found particularly relevant to my current situation is found in Isaiah Chapter 40, verse:31 But as I mentioned in the previous chapter, I have since augmented that verse with the 23rd psalm to reflect the additional support that I feel I have received from above.

LESSON 5: IT'S NOT YOUR FAULT

Cancer patients have a tendency to second guess the past. I know that I did. Why did this happen to me? What did I do wrong? But that kind of thinking does not help in your treatments or in the outcome. Getting cancer or any other serious disease is not your fault. You just have to know that these kinds of things happen in life, and your objective now is not to dwell on what might have been but on what is and can be. So I believe the best option is to get your plan in place and stick with it. Don't think about who or what is to blame in the past. Think about your actions going forward.

LESSON 6: YOU'VE GOT TO HAVE HOPE

There is a song in the musical Damn Yankees called "You've got to have heart" sung by the Washington baseball team in the locker room regarding their game with the Yankees. One line in the song goes "You've got to have hope; mustn't sit around and mope." And that is true in the fight against cancer or any other serious disease. You have got to hope that you will succeed. You have got to have hope that tomorrow will be better than today. You have got to have hope that the treatment will work. If you don't have hope in what you are doing, then the odds are that it will be a self-fulfilling prophecy and you will fail. If you have hope at least a certain satisfaction will come in doing all that you can.

I now wear a yellow Livestrong bracelet from the Lance Armstrong Foundation. Any time during the day that I feel that I am losing my confidence or feeling down about things, I take a look at the bracelet and it reminds me that I must have hope.

LESSON 7: DON'T HIDE IT

I found that talking about my situation was better than hiding it. As I mentioned earlier, we had a pretty good sized email base of family and friends that we would update after major events in my journey. I keep the Thursday church bible study group up to date on my progress. All of our local friends knew about my condition. We talked openly to other church members in the church coffee hour, a number of whom have had their own cancer experiences. One day I counted five church members coming in or going out of my oncologist's offices.

The one area of our lives that we did not talk about it much was to our real estate customers. As long as we were able to provide good service, we did not want to jeopardize relationships or business dealings by having customers worrying about my condition and questioning the service that I might be able to deliver. Some of our customers knew about my condition, but many of them did not. Those that did were supportive of us and always interested in my wellbeing.

LESSON 8: THE MIND VS THE BODY

My younger brother Jim has Parkinson's disease, which he developed shortly before I was diagnosed with cancer. His philosophy regarding the disease is that while his body is going through a physical transition over which he has little, if any control, his mind is still active. And as long as his mind is active, he can control his response to the disease. His belief about his ability to control the mental part of his life has stuck with me throughout my treatment. You can't worry about the how's and why's of cancer or any other disease, which is the physical side of things. What you can control is your response which is the mental side of things and which many would argue is most instrumental in your success in fighting the disease. His motto is, "I don't have Parkinson's. My body does." The same statement could be just as true with any other disease.

LESSON 9: KEEP A POSITIVE MENTAL ATTITUDE

Somewhere along my IBM career, I went to a seminar entitled "Success Through A Positive Mental Attitude." It focused on our own ability to determine what our mental attitude is going to be at any point in time and on our need to have a positive attitude every day. I mentioned earlier that people have commented to me about my positive attitude. I believe that, whether you are dealing with cancer or something else in your life, a daily positive attitude is one of the most important things that you can bring to the table and allows you to focus on what actions you can take to improve your situation.

LESSON 10: KNOW YOUR STUFF

I have found that the more you know about your specific cancer and your treatments, the better off you are, the better questions you can ask your oncologist and surgeon, and the more likely you are to understand their responses. As I mentioned earlier, I searched out a lot of information on the internet regarding colon cancer and its treatments. I am even signed for a service that distributes results of presentations from some of the annual meetings of the oncologists. And I download annual reports of the American Cancer Society. I have subscribed to Cure, a magazine dedicated to cancer education, and I pick up the pharma brochures on the various chemos that I take. I also get a lot of side information from the chemo nurses. It makes me feel good to know that I have a bit of the knowledge it takes to understand the cancer that I have and empowers me in handling my situation.

You can do the same sort of research with any condition that you are dealing with. Today there is basically no limit to the amount of information that one can obtain from the internet. Just make sure that it is current and not outdated. All too often I may be reading a cancer update and then notice that it is dated 2002. This information is probably not worth reading.

LESSON 11: TAKE CONTROL

When you have knowledge about your disease and its treatments, you have a chance to take control of your situation. Not that you are going to be your own doctor or surgeon, but that you are going to know what treatments you are on, what your treatment options are, what your treatment schedule is going to be, when your next scans are going to be scheduled and any other activities that might be necessary for your treatment. This is all part of the strategy to stick to your plan, to learn to control your disease and not let it control you.

LESSON 12: EXPECT THE UNEXPECTED

Things won't go as you have planned. Just when you think that things will be getting back to a more normal situation, you will probably get some unexpected news. The situation will have outwitted you again. So you need to expect surprises. That is why it is very important to have your plan in place. But you may need to adapt it to new conditions. There may be bumps along the road, but you can learn to deal with them. Expect the abnormal to be normal and you won't get discouraged when it happens.

LESSON 13: PLANNING FOR THE FUTURE

Planning events for some time in the future helps to take your mind off of the problems with your current situation and provide optimism for the future. And that is a positive thing. If you are actively thinking about an event next week, next month or even next year, you have less time to think about your current problems. It almost doesn't matter what it is; a dinner out, a trip to a nearby city for a play, or a vacation trip to Europe. Having events on the calendar will get you to thinking about them and may even increase your motivation to "make it to the date." And once reaching the event successfully, you can then make more plans for the future. The more time you spend on planning non-medical related events and the less time you spend thinking about your disease, the better off you will be.

LESSON: 14: A DAY AT A TIME

It may sound a little cliché to say it, but you have to take life's journey a day at a time. Getting stage IV colon cancer, or any serious cancer or disease for that matter, is not a good thing. But with the treatments available today you can, hopefully, hang on for a long time. That's what I hope happens to me. So what you have to do is take the day you have today and make the best of it. You can't do anything more about yesterday and you can have a plan for tomorrow, but today is the day that you can actually make something happen. Focus your energy on today.

LESSON 15: KEEP YOUR SENSE OF HUMOR

No matter what you may be going through in your life, it helps to have a sense of humor. I have found that even in the most serious of situations a little humor can often break the ice and take the edge off of things. Tell a joke now and then. I think that people with a sense of humor probably enjoy their lives more than people without one. It does not take any more time in the day to laugh a bit. And it is probably good medicine for what ails you.

LESSON 16: PLAY THE HAND YOU ARE DEALT

This one also may be a little bit trite, but I believe that it applies to many situations. You have to live your own life with all of its ups and downs. You are not living your brother's life, your neighbor's life, or your best friend's life. You are living your own life. You have been given certain skills just the same as I have. But your skills are different than mine. And the aspects of your life will be different as well. And so the hand that you play will be different. That does not mean that it will be any easier or any tougher just that it will be different. And so what you do with it will be different as well.

But life is not like duplicate bridge, where the playing of the hand is measured against the standard of a group. You are the only one who knows how well you are playing it. Make sure that you give it your best effort. You may be able to play it better than you think. And above all use the skills that you were given; don't waste them.

Epilogue

So this brings us up to date with the current status of things in the life and times of Papa Vark. A lot of interesting things have happened so far, and with any luck there is a lot more to come. I hope that you have enjoyed reading about the journey as much as I have enjoyed narrating it to you.

My wife and I live in a part of Princeton that has a lot of birds. When I first started being called a Vark, my daughter, Kelly, took a yellow pad and wrote down some instructions for daily living for me that I have scotch-taped to the window ledge of my home office. I still find them useful to this day. You might find them useful as well. They are as follows:

Vark Around
Watch the Birds
Work on Nap

And so there you have it.

Author's Notes

I started thinking about this book at the time that I published my previous book *On The Far Side Of The Curve* the end of 2009. There were many stories and anecdotes about my life that I did not include in that book that I thought would be lost if I did not make the effort to write them down and incorporate them in the new book that you are holding in your hand. And I have worked on this new book off and on over the last two years.

I am indebted to a number of people for their support and comments on my manuscript. First of all, to my wife and caregiver, Patricia, who has been a sounding-board throughout. Then, to my children, Scott and Kelly, and Scott's wife, Cristina, who gave their approval to my efforts. To my older brother, Dean, who had provided some thoughts on our early years before he passed away this past August. To my brothers, Allen and Jim, and to Barbara Fox, who read the latest draft from cover to cover and uncovered numerous errors in my writing. And, finally, to a select group of friends; Tim and Linda Henry, and Jack Taylor who gave me frequent guidance and encouragement on the structure and content of the book. I thank them all and believe that this is a much better book because of their input and their able assistance. Any errors that remain are mine alone.

In Memoriam

Wayne passed away before this book could be published. He fought his cancer bravely and with dignity for over eight years. We miss him dearly and we know that he set an example for which we can all be proud.

Pat, Scott and Kelly